Numb Toes and Aching Soles

Numb Toes and Aching Soles:
Coping With Peripheral Neuropathy

JOHN A. SENNEFF

MEDPRESS
Halifax, Nova Scotia

Published by
MedPress
PO Box 81
Halifax, Nova Scotia
B3J 2L4 Canada

Library of Congress Catalog Card Number: 99-62350

ISBN (pbk.): 978-0-9781820-0-7
ISBN (hrdbk): 978-0-9781820-1-4

This text is printed on acid-free paper.

Printed in the United States of America

10 9 8

To those suffering from the pain of
peripheral neuropathy in its most cruel forms,
that they may find help and hope in these pages.

Contents

Foreword

With *Numb Toes and Aching Soles: Coping with Peripheral Neuropathy*, John Senneff has created an admirable and valuable resource for the many individuals who experience and suffer from pain related to peripheral neuropathy.

As background, peripheral neuropathies are a common, but complex group of disorders for neurologists and other physicians. While peripheral neuropathy may affect the smallest of children, it is especially common in middle and late adulthood, with an estimated prevalence of three to four percent. About one-half of peripheral neuropathies are related to complications from diabetes mellitus. The other half are a mixed bag, and many of these are idiopathic or cryptogenic, meaning no definitive cause can be found to explain the peripheral nerve injury. My experience and reports from other academic medical centers suggest that 10–25% of peripheral neuropathies remain unexplained even after thorough evaluations in university-based neurology departments.

While the cardinal features of peripheral neuropathy are loss of sensation and weakness—most frequently in the feet and hands—several common forms of peripheral

neuropathy, in what seems paradoxical, produce significant pain and discomfort. Burning, stinging, throbbing,
tingling, stabbing, aching, and shooting pains are all possible. In truth, just about any unpleasant sensation may
be experienced by individuals with peripheral neuropathy.
Foot pain is a frequent problem in diabetic neuropathy
and is present in 70–80 percent of idiopathic neuropathies. This book's purpose is to provide guidance and
comfort for those of you who suffer from neuropathic pain.

Early chapters of John's book are devoted to traditional or conventional treatments for neuropathic pain.
Many of these treatments have demonstrated effectiveness in carefully designed studies of patients with neuropathic pain. These agents are typically the starting-
point of therapy for physicians who care for patients with
painful peripheral neuropathy. Later chapters discuss alternative remedies as well as experimental agents still
under investigation.

First, a word regarding alternative therapy. There is a
general tendency for physicians to frown upon alternative treatments (herbal medicine, vitamin and mineral
supplements, etc.) because they have not undergone rigorous study according to accepted scientific standards.
Still, I would stress that management of neuropathic
pain is a difficult business, and by no means do conventional treatments benefit all patients. It is my practice to
allow patients significant latitude when it comes to alternative therapies, as long as I do not perceive any dan-
ger in what is being used.

In general, I caution patients to avoid megadoses of

any agent and to be wary of nutritionists or auxiliary caregivers who suggest taking large amounts of some substance on a regular basis. I also caution patients about alternative therapies that are exorbitant in cost or in claims of effectiveness. With those caveats in mind, alternative therapies are generally not harmful (to you or your pocketbook), and may even make you more comfortable. I certainly have neuropathy patients who responded poorly to a long list of conventional medications and later found some relief with alternative agents. I admit to keeping a list of anecdotal success stories from patients who swear by alternative or homemade remedies. I even admit to making suggestions from this list when I encounter a refractory patient who has not responded to or could not tolerate a variety of conventional agents, either individually or in combination. In the arena of pain management, we physicians can learn as much from you as you can from us.

Finally, I feel that some words of optimism are in order. Although finding an effective treatment with acceptable side effects can be challenging, I firmly believe that a large majority of you with neuropathic pain will benefit from one form of therapy or another. The discomfort may not vanish completely, but you will be more comfortable and functional, and life won't seem so dreadful anymore. But please be patient. It generally takes several weeks to determine whether or not an individual medication is helpful. Furthermore, choosing an agent largely remains a trial-and-error proposition. We physicians really cannot predict with any accuracy which patient will respond to which agent. So work with your caregiver and try to understand that if initial treatment approaches are not successful, this does not mean that your doctor does not take your symptoms seriously or is incompetent. You may be surprised to find an effective therapy just around the corner.

Lastly, join the Neuropathy Association. This is a wonderful patient based organization built around an alliance between neuropathy patients and physicians. The Neuropathy Association's mission is to support and educate patients and physicians, advocate for patient interests, and promote research in the cause and treatment of peripheral neuropathy. The Association can be reached by telephone at 1-800-247-6968 or on the Internet at http://www.neuropathy.org/neuropathy. I wish you the best and hope you find John's book instructive and enlightening.

Gil I. Wolfe, M.D.
Department of Neurology
University of Texas Southwestern Medical Center
Dallas, Texas

Preface

I have had peripheral neuropathy (PN) for more than ten years. It was not until quite recently, though, I discovered that was the name for my affliction.

In the mid '80s I began to experience numbness in my toes and tingling, prickling, burning sensations which seemed, at different times, to radiate all over my feet. It bothered me particularly after I jogged. Also I became aware of a growing deadening of the soles and a much greater sensitivity to touch on the tops and sides of my feet. Even though there wasn't much feeling on the bottoms it really hurt to walk barefoot over hard surfaces, particularly if the surfaces were uneven. Talk about a strange bag of contradictory symptoms!

An electric foot massager helped a little—but only when using it. I didn't do much else at the time other than to ease up on the jogging. Eventually that had to be given up altogether, which really bothered me because I enjoyed running.

Various people had different ideas concerning my problem. One or another would say it must be due to foot pronation or a chemical imbalance, or maybe vitamin deficiency, poor circulation, or perhaps it was due to two herniated discs which were surgically fused. Nobody mentioned the possibility of peripheral neuropathy. Not even, when my condition worsened and I sought professional help, did either of two orthopedic specialists to whom I went, or either of two acupuncturists, a podiatrist, a reflexologist, or even a neurologist who ran a cursory nerve conduction test and pronounced me fine! Two of these professionals dismissed the problem—and me— by prescribing orthotic devices to be worn in my shoes.

I didn't hear the word "neuropathy" until about two years ago. At that time I started going to a physical therapist for muscle toning; he mentioned it as a possibility. However, the doctor of "sports medicine" with whom he was associated waved off the notion—without testing or suggesting tests. She strongly urged me to go through a series of acupuncture sessions she could perform which she was quite sure could help my problem—whatever it might be. They didn't and were $75 a pop, unreimbursed by insurance; I stopped after two.

I then began to experience nearly constant pain every time I walked or even stood for long. As for going across a parking lot or through a big store with concrete floors like Home Depot—forget it! Sometimes I would just look at my feet and think I'd be better off without those dogs. I finally decided to go to an internist I knew, hoping he could point me in the right direction. After listening to my symptoms and doing some preliminary testing he said he suspected peripheral neuropathy. He immediately arranged with a well-qualified neurologist for further evaluation. This neurologist's examination, which was much more thorough than that performed by the first one, confirmed the diagnosis. He and the internist established a regimen of medication for me which helped a good deal—along with some vitamins and herbs I'm taking. I still don't have the pain completely licked but I'm a whole lot better than I was.

Since getting a grasp on my own situation and talking to many others, I've been amazed at the general lack of knowledge concerning peripheral neuropathy—this bizarre affliction which so few people know by name but which so many endure. One only has to look at postings on Internet bulletin boards, forums and news groups to realize there are many with pain and other physical complaints which suggest peripheral neuropathy but who either don't know what they have or don't know how to deal with it. And in many instances their professional caretakers don't seem to have a clue either. (The point was made at an American Medical Association—AMA—panel discussion in New York in July 1997 that some 40 to 67% of pain cases are misdiagnosed, preventing successful treatment.)

PN victims seeking answers are not going to get much help from general medical books covering diseases, disorders, medical testing or treatments. I went to the medical section of a large national chain book store and looked at the biggest books with the most pages on these subjects. A good third did not mention peripheral neuropathy at all! Except for one (*Merck Manual,* 16th Edition), they were largely useless in describing the disorder or commenting on tests and treatments. In fact the only books I've come across specifically directed to the subject were written for the medical profession and are expensive. (A frustrated lady recently lamented on an Internet forum that she had "yet to find a book on PN and had been looking for three years.")

The following excerpt from a PNer[1] which appeared on an Internet bulletin board illustrates what too often is happening in the real world. She had developed leg cramps, which in her case were an early warning of "Restless Legs Syndrome" (RLS), a malady frequently associated with peripheral neuropathy. Her doctor had dismissed her complaints, saying she just "needed some calcium":

"Now I know that this was RLS and the early signs of PN. My Neurologist agrees, and offers little comment other than reaffirming that many PN patients either were or are RLS sufferers. The tragedy of this is that so many of us are now comparing stories and seeing that we had early warning signs that were ignored . . . either by ourselves or by our physicians. How can that be? I told myself that my legs were overtired from clomping around work in high heels . . . that, like the doctor said, all women have leg cramps at one time or another. I felt like a big baby complaining about my feet hurting. Plus I also felt guilty about taking up his time

---

[1] I'm usually going to use the term "PNers" in this book to say who we are—not always but most times. I like it because it's short and has an elite ring to it—like either we're members of a very exclusive club or that we've all been retired from some honored combat group. (Combat is what this feels like at times; unfortunately we're still on active duty.) Besides, "sufferers" sounds self-pitying. "Victims" sounds like we were hit by a truck. "Patients" sounds like we were hit by a truck and are now recovering at the hospital. And if I used "afflictees," as I first thought to do, you wouldn't have to be told I was a lawyer!

with something that I didn't understand or couldn't even describe. 'My feet feel like there are creepy crawlers on them' didn't arouse his curiosity, 'my feet jerk and jump' got a blank stare into space. 'My feet cramp and my toes strain' bingo . . . he recognized that symptom, take two Quinnam [quinine tablets]before bedtime and don't worry about it! Sadly, as I look back, this set the stage for my dealing with doctors for PN. I continued to accept the mis-diagnoses, lack of concern, shrug of shoulders, and pats on the back while being pushed out the door. After all, it must be me that's CRAZY . . . it couldn't be the four doctors! So here I am, a physical mess, wishing I knew then what I know now. I'd like to drag my soapbox up to the main inter-section of town and shout the message out. There are thou-sands of us PN people out here who don't know the WHY's and HOW's of this disease. There is no standard or proven treatment plan, we don't know how far it will advance, we don't even have neurologists who agree on the symptoms or medications. Surely someone in the medical training field should be telling the new doctors about these symptoms, teaching them to LISTEN to what the patients are saying, to explore the possibility that maybe, just MAYBE, they aren't making idle complaints . . . maybe, just MAYBE, there may actually be a progressive, disabling disease at work. OK, OK, I'll put my soapbox back in the garage for now. But, it re-ally makes me mad that the majority of posts on the BB say the same thing . . . by the time they were diagnosed it was too late! Isn't that a tragedy! I'm so mad I'm gonna go eat some ice cream!!"

After reading various stories like this and thinking more about my own case I decided to learn as much as possible about peripheral neuropathy and what could be done about it, then share with others the information I had gathered. To this end I've spent well over a thousand hours on the Internet and elsewhere studying the huge amount of information pertaining to PN and related subjects, sifting out what seemed most relevant, helpful and interesting for this book. I've also spoken with neurologists, other practitioners and people in the medical industry from all over the country concerning a number of subjects treated here.

My first purpose is to explain in non-technical terms what peripheral neuropathy is, how you get it and what it does to you. This is meant not only to let uninformed PNers know more about their malady but to give family and friends some appreciation of what their PNer is up against.

The real meat in the book, though, is treatments. Everything I could find on this most important (to the PNer) subject I thought would be helpful is covered. Treatments currently being prescribed—traditional (both conventional and aggressive) as well as so-called alternative medical approaches, together with vitamins and other nutritional aids—are all dealt with in depth. Additionally a number of new drugs and other compounds now being investigated, which might finally provide total relief from peripheral neuropathic pain and from other PN effects, are discussed in detail. One of these might even prove to be the long sought cure!

I've also included many comments from various Internet bulletin boards, forums and news groups concerning experiences people have had with therapies discussed in this book, both with regard to their efficacy and their side effects. The idea is to give you a sense of what different people think about the medications and other things they've tried. After all, this book is not meant to be a medical text hypothesizing the outcome of various treatments in the abstract. It's a guide for real PN victims suffering real pains or other problems and wondering, desperately sometimes, what in fact has helped (or hurt) others.

To me these patient comments are among the most valuable parts of this book. Please consider when you review them, though, that each of us is different and that what works for this one or affects that one won't necessarily produce similar outcomes for others. Even more importantly, the people who are making these comments are *those with peripheral neuropathy, not doctors treating it*. You should not regard any of these remarks as medical opinions on which you can rely. However, they *do* have the force of personal experience behind them and they certainly can serve as starting points for talking over various possible therapies with your doctor. Who knows, if the doctor is open minded—and I hope for your sake that's the case—maybe even he or she will learn or be led to something new.

There is also a chapter on special considerations for diabetic and HIV-related neuropathies. An amazingly high percentage of people in these two groups suffer from this disorder and have unique problems of their own.

Finally, I've laid out some ideas I've come across on how to enjoy a better quality of life if you do have PN. Ideas on what to wear, what to eat or not eat, how to sleep, whether and to what extent exercise is appropriate and for some, just how to get through each day.

As an *apologia,* my principal qualification for writing this book (apart from my willingness to devour the subject to the last byte) is that, as a PNer, I have had personal experience with the kind of pain peripheral neuropathy can deliver—pain that can claw at you and then let go for awhile only to come back and tear away more savagely than before. Consequently, I can empathize with others who have PN and think I can bring insights that a medical professional does not have who has only studied it from a distance and who doesn't know how it *really* feels. One woman on an Internet bulletin board put it this way: "I love being able to say the word 'burn' and know that you understand I'm not talking about 'burning feet' but 'BU-U-U-RNING Feet'!"

*   *   *

I strongly urge people who think they may have peripheral neuropathy, and their caretakers, to join the **Neuropathy Association**. It's a non-profit organization with over 14,000 members, all in the same boat. The Association publishes a newsletter and sponsors over 100 support groups. You will gain much by being a member! As Dr. Wolfe said in the foreword, the Association can be reached at 1-800-247-6968 or at their web site: www.neuropathy.org.

Various products I've come across are mentioned which might be helpful to PNers. I have absolutely no financial interest in any of the companies which produce them. I have personally tried only a few and I certainly do not warrant the safety or effectiveness of any of them. My sole purpose is to bring them to your attention for your or your attending physician's consideration.

A final note. There is no intention here to give medical advice. I am a retired lawyer with peripheral neuropathy, not a practicing doctor prescribing for it. To me that's an advantage because I can write from a different point of view. If you have symptoms which suggest peripheral neuropathy you should go to a qualified physician as soon as possible for a thorough evaluation and proposed course of treatment. The sections that deal with existing medications and procedures are meant only to inform you what some doctors are now prescribing for their patients and what some PNers are experiencing. There is *no* intention on my part to recommend *any* particular therapy or approach to treatment. You should rely solely on your doctor concerning the most appropriate treatment for YOU.

Acknowledgments

I owe a debt of deep gratitude to a number of people in completing this book. Included are some of the finest neurologists in the country with expertise in peripheral nerve disorders. These doctors, many of whom are on faculties of major teaching institutions, amazed me by their willingness to spend as much time as they did poring over earlier drafts. In doing so they demonstrated a genuine compassion and concern for those for whom this book is written.

The detailed comments of these doctors helped immeasurably in making the book better and far more useful than it would have been otherwise. At the same time I want to make clear that any errors, omissions or matters of misplaced emphasis which may remain are solely my responsibility, not theirs.

Here are the neurologists who were so helpful:

Dr. Anthony Amato, University of Texas Health Science Center, San Antonio, Texas;

Dr. Arthur K. Asbury, Van Meter Professor of Neurology Emeritus, University of Pennsylvania School of Medicine, Philadelphia, Pennsylvania;

Dr. Richard L. Barbano, Assistant Professor of
Neurology, University of Rochester School of Medicine and Dentistry, Rochester, New York;

Dr. David A. Greenberg, Professor and Vice-Chairman of Neurology, University of Pittsburgh School of
Medicine, Pittsburgh, Pennsylvania;

Dr. James H. Halsey, Professor of Neurology, Columbia University College of Physicians and Surgeons,
New York City, New York;

Dr. Laurence J. Kinsella, Chief, Division of Neurology, Mt. Sinai Medical Center, Cleveland, Ohio;

Dr. Richard A. Lewis, Professor of Neurology and
Associate Chair, Wayne State University School of
Medicine, Detroit, Michigan;

Dr. Avertano Noronha, Associate Professor of Clinical Neurology, University of Chicago, Chicago, Illinois

Dr. Shin J. Oh, Professor of Neurology, University of
Alabama, Birmingham, Alabama;

Dr. Anibal F. Prentice, Neurologist, Kansas City,
Missouri;

Dr. A. Gordon Smith, Assistant Professor of Neurology, University of Utah School of Medicine, Salt
Lake City, Utah;

Dr. Joseph Wilner, Neurologist, Englewood, New
Jersey; and

Dr. Gil I. Wolfe, Professor of Neurology, University of
Texas Southwestern Medical Center at Dallas, Texas.

I also want to thank Rosemary Waggener, Bill Cracken
and Jim Miller, members of our Neuropathy Association

support group in San Antonio, Texas. They helped greatly in providing valuable comments on the manuscript from the patient's point of view. Jim, our fearless leader, has shown that in another life he could be copy editor for a major New York publishing house. (In this one he was an aeronautical engineer, now retired.)

Finally I want to thank my wife, Beth, for her many probing questions and intelligent comments on all the drafts she looked at. (Beth wouldn't like the previous sentence because it ends with a preposition.) She has been a true and wonderful help-mate all the way. (And by saying this I hope I can coax her into going over the manuscript one more time. After note—she did, bless her.)

Chapter 1

What It Is and How You Get It

Millions in this country and elsewhere have peripheral neuropathy in different forms and to various degrees. The number usually cited in the U.S. is two million. Yet a study of its incidence just among specific population groups, for example among people with diabetes or with HIV infections, would suggest a much larger number.

It can strike any age group in any social or cultural strata.[1] Many, perhaps most, victims do not realize what ails their aching soles and numb toes, as well as their tingling fingers, throbbing hands or weakening muscles. The shame of this is that without early action based on knowledge of their afflictions, the pain and other symptoms experienced by these sufferers almost invariably

---

[1] Older people are particularly at risk. The May 1998 issue of the *Women's Health Advocate* claimed that as many as *20%* of older Americans have PN! (No study or other documentation was advanced for this statistic.)

gets worse. Moreover, their neuropathies often tend to advance in their bodies, causing more and more areas to be affected. Another problem is that if attention is delayed certain neuropathies can become more difficult to treat.

Peripheral Neuropathy Explained

Perhaps because it's poorly understood and not commonly discussed, peripheral neuropathy is sometimes called the "silent disease" (though it has company using this tag!). Yet it affects more people than rheumatoid arthritis—a much better known ailment—with just as severe consequences in its worst form.

To start with, it should be understood PN is not really a disease at all. Rather it's a **complex** of **disorders** in the **peripheral nervous system** resulting from damage to the nerves' protective coating or from damage to the nerves themselves.

Our peripheral nervous system is made up of nerve fibers bundled together in nerve trunks. They run from the brain and spinal cord (which make up the **central nervous system**) to other parts of our body. The fibers are shielded by a coating or membrane called the **myelin sheath**. Like wires protected by insulation, the coated fibers carry "electrical" impulses from **receptors** located in internal organs, muscles and skin, back to our brain through our spinal cord. When an injury to our peripheral nerves or their protective coating occurs which interferes with the transmission of impulses from these receptors, one of two things (or sometimes both) occurs depending on the receptors and nerve fibers involved. Either the brain simply acknowledges and registers the abnormal transmission as pain or some other unpleasant sensation,[2] or it prompts a response back to the muscle or organ from which the original impulse emanated. In the latter case the response may result in decreased muscle movement or changes in organ functioning.

Peripheral neuropathy (particularly sensory neuropathy—more on that later) seems in most cases to initially occur at the extremities of the longest nerves farthest from the spinal cord and brain.[3] Consequently the feet, being at the end of the line, are usually the first to be hit. Frequently the hands are next. Over time the affliction can spread to ankles, legs and arms if the underlying cause is not addressed.

Types

Most of the disorders dealt with in this book are called **"polyneuropathies."** This means that they are multiple and usually (but not always) symmetric, affecting both

---

[2] Of course if the nerve is destroyed the brain may not recognize pain or any other sensation.

[3] One neurologist, a specialist in cancer-related neuropathies, pointed out to me that in some cases, for example, occasionally with diabetic or with paraneoplastic—tumor related—sensory neuropathy, the spinal cord itself may be directly affected, sparing the longest nerves.

feet, for example, or both hands, in the same way. A term often used to describe this condition is "**distal symmetrical polyneuropathy**." In contrast "**mononeuropathy**" refers to the injury of a single nerve such as in **carpal tunnel syndrome**, where only one hand and wrist may be affected, or **Bell's palsy**, involving a single nerve to facial muscles.

Other neuropathy classifications are based on whether the sensory, motor or autonomic nerve fibers are involved. Damage to **sensory fibers**, concerned with feeling and touching, results either in abnormal *paresthesias* (sensations) such as tingling, numbness, electrical shocks, or in outright pain. Damage to **motor fibers**, which are responsible for voluntary movements such as fist clenching, may result in bodily changes such as muscle weakness or atrophy, or cramps and spasms. Damage to **autonomic fibers**, which affect involuntary or semi-voluntary functions such as control of internal organs, can cause such changes as decreased ability to sweat, loss in blood pressure (with or without dizziness), constipation, bowel and bladder problems, and sexual dysfunction.

Somewhat rarer neuropathies and attendant complications include:

Chronic Inflammatory Demyelinating Polyneuropathy (CIDP is a chronic autoimmune disorder— the immune system itself is attacking the myelin sheath—and is characterized by muscle weakness and burning sensations);

Guillain-Barre syndrome (GBS is also autoimmune,

oftentimes resulting in paralysis of the legs, arms and breathing muscles);

Charcot-Marie-Tooth disease (CMT is a complex of hereditary nerve disorders of various types frequently involving the myelin sheath); and

"Restless Legs Syndrome" (RLS is a **complication** of neuropathy—as well as of iron deficiency anemia—manifested by creeping, crawling sensations accompanied by motor restlessness, most often experienced at night).

The Neuropathy Association (mentioned in the Foreword and Preface) publishes an excellent booklet written by Dr. Norman Latov (Professor of Neurology at Columbia University) and Mary Ann Donovan (President of the Association) as a primer on peripheral neuropathy. It lists a number of neuropathic disorders in terms of whether they are "acquired" or "inherited."

Symptoms and Effects

Symptoms of **sensory neuropathies**, which may gradually occur over many months, often include numbness of the affected members, burning, tingling sensations, "electric" shocks, aching pain and extreme sensitivity to touch.

Motor neuropathies frequently result in weakness in the feet, ankles, hands and wrists. Diarrhea, lightheadedness or sexual dysfunction are some of the possible consequences of **autonomic neuropathies**. In severe cases involving these neuropathies, activities such as walking normally and sleeping may be nearly impossible.

In rare situations even respiratory failure or paralysis may occur with certain neuropathies such as **Guillain-Barre syndrome.**

Causes

There are said to be more than 100 causes of peripheral neuropathy. **Diabetes** is considered the most common, at least in the United States.[4] It is variously estimated that 30 to 65% of people with diabetes have PN to some degree. In this group it is especially prevalent among those having particular difficulty in controlling their blood glucose levels and/or those having high lipid levels (cholesterol and triglycerides), those over 40 and among smokers.

PN also is said to cause pain for up to one-third of people with **AIDS** or **HIV**. In fact it is thought to be the most frequent neurologic disorder associated with HIV infection, typically occurring in the later stages of the disease.

Various **toxins** and **metallic poisons** (such as arsenic, lead and mercury), certain **chemicals** (especially solvents and some insecticides), excessive **alcohol** in-

---

[4] A neurologist up on these matters told me leprosy is the most common cause of PN world wide.

take, **vitamin deficiencies** (particularly B12) or **vitamin excesses** (B6), **nutritional imbalances**, and a number of **drugs** used to treat HIV infections and AIDS can all cause peripheral neuropathy. It can also result from **kidney failure**, **liver disease**, **rheumatoid arthritis**, **abnormal blood proteins**, **cancer**[5] (and even **cancer chemotherapy**), **leukemia** and **shingles**.

Certain **repetitive activities** such as typing can also be the cause of some neuropathies. **Carpal tunnel syndrome** is one example. This is a so-called **entrapment neuropathy**—a condition resulting from a nerve lesion at a point where the nerve is confined to a narrow passageway. Another instance of entrapment neuropathy is where restrictive clothing compresses a nerve called the

---

[5] One neurologist advised me that a paraneoplastic (tumor-related) neuropathy could be an early sign of cancer. It comes about in this way: when the body's immune system detects a cancerous tumor it pulls out all the stops in attacking it. However, the immune system in its fury sometimes fails to recognize the true target and may attack peripheral nerves instead. The paraneoplastic neuropathy resulting from the nerve damage thus indicates a cancerous tumor may be present.

An interesting study reported in the July 1998 issue of the journal, *Archives of Neurology*, suggests, at least by implication, a possibly different kind of link between **idiopathic** neuropathy and cancer. Fifty-one patients (42 men and 9 women with a mean age of 64.5 years) without any identified cause of their neuropathies were observed over a period of time. More than a third developed cancer *after* the onset of their neuropathies, the cancers being diagnosed at a mean interval of 27.9 months following neuropathic onset. The cancer was in the liver in 4, the bladder in 3, the lymph nodes in 3, the prostate gland in 2, the lungs in 2, the breast in 1, the pancreas in 1, the sublingual gland in 1 and the bone in 1. The investigators of the study did note two earlier studies had shown fewer instances of post-neuropathy cancer occuring than had their own.

lateral femoral cutaneous nerve which runs from the groin to the upper thigh.[6]

A tendency toward peripheral neuropathy can also be **inherited**. A family history of the disorder increases the likelihood. In a different twist on inherited susceptibility, a study done in France in 1995, reported in the November 1995 issue of *Alcohol and Alcoholism*, suggested a relationship between a history of alcoholism in a *father* and peripheral neuropathy in his alcoholic offspring. Ninety alcoholics, some with neuropathies and some without, were included in the study. The investigators found neuropathies occurred in alcoholics five times as often when the father was an alcoholic himself than when he was not. (Unfortunately, the study did not consider the incidence of PN in the alcoholic fathers, raising the obvious question whether perhaps it was the PN itself which was inherited rather than a greater disposition to neuropathy simply because of the paternal alcoholism. P.S. I hope you follow me here!)

The publication *Bio Medical Frontiers* reports that the cause of one third of all neuropathies is unknown—mine included. These cryptogenic disorders are called "**idiopathic**." Some clinicians believe many of these unexplained cases are really genetic in origin.

Incidentally, I discovered that not only does my neuropathy have a name—idiopathic—it has a number. Under the International Classification of Diseases—a

---

[6] There is some evidence that people with neuropathy are prone to new nerve damage in knee and elbow areas, representing pressure points in the body. It's suggested by some practitioners that PNers refrain from prolonged kneeling or elbow leaning because of this.

world-wide system which groups related diseases and procedures for reporting statistical information—idiopathic neuropathy is code 356.8. A word of advice: if you happen to be idiopathic and are ever doing a slow shuffle down the street, having a particularly bad day with your PN, and somebody annoyingly asks what's wrong with you, you can be sure they won't stay around too long if you say "I've got the 356.8 disease."

Evaluation and Testing

1. Purpose

Obviously if one has suspicious symptoms, the first reason to see a physician is to determine whether peripheral neuropathy, or some other malady, is present.

If a physician suspects neuropathy, thorough evaluation and testing may give clues to the probable cause and may suggest a course of treatment. For example, it is important in determining treatment to know whether the injury is to the nerve fibers themselves or to the myelin sheath covering them. Also the severity of the injury can be established through tests. Dr. Peter J. Dyck at the Mayo Clinic in Rochester, Minnesota (editor of the treatise, *Peripheral Neuropathy*, Dyck & Thomas, W. B. Saunders, 1993, regarded as the medical "bible" with respect to PN) has been quoted as saying:

"Neurologists need to judge severity of neuropathy in order to:

Ascertain the degree of neurologic impairment.

Decide on how comprehensive an evaluation for underlying cause is justified.

Come to a conclusion about whether therapy should be begun, altered, or stopped.

Make inferences about outlook.

Decide whether a given therapy is efficacious."

A search for **reversible causes** is always an important part of this process. For example, it might be determined that a certain toxin in the blood, or a deficiency of vitamin B12, is the culprit. This then would suggest a treatment approach.

Even when the cause of the primary neuropathy has been established, medical practitioners will sometimes wish to determine whether another disorder may be involved and co-exist with the primary neuropathy. This is particularly true where there is a frequent relationship between the two. For example, a person with diabetic PN might well have carpal tunnel syndrome or another entrapment neuropathy (mentioned above) which needs to be treated separately.

2. Procedures

Before any testing is undertaken the physician will (or should) carefully go over the patient's **medical history**. This would include asking about symptoms, medications currently being taken or taken during the last several years, any past or present exposure to conditions that could possibly cause or aggravate a neuropathy (such as paints or various toxins), and social habits frequently associated with PN such as smoking or drinking. You as the patient should take thoughtful time to write down and document as much as you can matters concerning your condition (when it occurred, symptoms, any contributing factor you can think of, etc.) before you see a physician so that your time together may prove as productive as possible.

The doctor will likely determine first whether **ankle jerks** can be induced, the absence of which may indicate PN. Also testing sensations in the feet, hands and other regions with a **sharp pointed object** will disclose different levels of sensitivity which could indicate neuropathy.

Loss of vibratory sensation can be assessed by applying a **128 Hz tuning fork** over the great toe. Those who have sensory neuropathy may only feel a buzzing for several seconds versus 10 seconds or more for those with normal sensation. Another quick test often used in doctors' offices involves a **nylon filament** mounted on a small wand. To determine if the patient can feel pressure a standardized force is delivered by the wand to certain areas of the foot.

Blood and **urine** tests are commonly employed to test for vitamin deficiencies (e.g., vitamin B12) and toxic elements which could possibly cause neuropathy.

Based on the initial evaluation the primary care physician may decide to refer the patient to a neurologist for further testing. **Nerve conduction** studies conducted by this specialist can usually confirm neuropathy and differentiate injury to the nerve fibers from injury to the myelin sheath. In these studies round metallic electrodes are placed on the skin and over the nerves at various points on the body. The electrodes constitute anodes and cathodes, and a low intensity electric current is introduced to stimulate the nerves. The velocity at which the resulting electric impulses are transmitted through the nerves is determined when images of the impulses are projected on an oscilloscope or computer screen. If a particular response is **slower** or **weaker** than normal, damage to the myelin sheath is implied. If the **height** of the response's **amplitude** is low, damage to the nerve axon is implied. Most neuropathies are caused by axonal damage rather than demyelination.[7]

Electromyography (EMG) tests involve the insertion of fine needles into muscle tissues. The needles, which serve as electrodes, provide information about the muscle itself and indicate how well it is supplied by nerve. The EMG can help differentiate nerve disorders from primary muscle conditions. (Some patients have difficulty tolerating EMGs. Could simply seeing needles coming their way have anything to do with it?)

A fairly new patient-friendly device called the **Tacticon** is being sold by Flocare Medical (800-804-6358). It's a seven ounce hand held tool with seven probes of various diameters held against the skin. According to the company, if the patient is unable to differentiate among the probes, nerve ending damage is indicated. Advan-

---

[7] A neurologist told me that some of his patients **with** peripheral neuropathy had **normal** nerve conduction tests and that others who **did not** have PN had **abnormal** readings! He stressed that the examining neurologist cannot rely solely on such tests but rather needs to make a clinical diagnosis based on a meticulous examination of the patient and a careful review of the patient's history.

tages claimed are that it can be used by general practitioners for initial screening and is inexpensive compared to conventional equipment. There are various other screening devices commercially available.

A **lumbar puncture** or **spinal tap** may be used in some cases to identify the presence of an autoimmune disorder such as Guillain-Barre syndrome (GBS) or chronic inflammatory demyelinating polyneuropathy (CIDP). This involves the insertion of a long thin needle into the spinal canal to sample fluid and measure pressure. The procedure also may be used to test for multiple sclerosis or other inflammatory disease of the central nervous system if this type of disorder is suspected.

Occasionally **magnetic resonance imaging** (MRI) is used if there is a question of arthritic changes in the spine causing compression of spinal nerve roots.

Nerve biopsies, involving the surgical removal and examination of nerve tissue, are sometimes performed when a diagnosis based on the foregoing tests remains in doubt or when the disorder appears particularly severe.[8] As one neurologist pointed out to me, a nerve biopsy provides the only opportunity to directly visualize the damaged nerve.

Unfortunately, though, many people report greater pain or discomfort following this procedure than they had before the surgery. Consequently, most practitioners limit nerve biopsies to situations where there is a good chance a **treatable cause** of the neuropathy can be

---

[8] Less commonly, **skin** biopsies are sometimes performed to assess the **density** of nerve fibers.

identified. An example is where the neuropathy might
be due to **vasculitis**—an inflammation of blood vessels
in the nerve—and be associated with a rheumatological
disease such as lupus or rheumatoid arthritis. One
neurologist told me that a nerve biopsy, in fact, is the
only certain way to make such a determination.

Chapter 2

Peripheral Neuropathy Pain

Peripheral neuropathy creates a number of unpleasant problems for many PNers, depending on the particular type involved. As noted, these may include numbness, muscle weakness, movement impairment, loss of balance or position sense, breathing difficulties and sexual dysfunction, to name a few. The worst problems facing most PNers, however, have to do with pain, particularly pain resulting from **sensory** neuropathies.

This neuropathic pain comes in all shapes and sizes. It can be dull, diffuse and persistent; sharp, stabbing and intermittent; or constantly burning. At different times it can seem to be a combination of all of these. At its worse the pain feels like it's taken on a life of its own, unrelenting and interminable. In fact it can become like a disease itself, wearing the sufferer down as a result of anxiety, depression and loss of sleep.

There appear to be both **physical** and **psychological** aspects to PN pain. The first is based, according to most experts, on an alteration of electrical signals that are formed by sensors in various parts of the body and transmitted through the peripheral nervous system to the brain. The psychological aspect is based on how the victim perceives the altered signals and reacts to them as a result of attitude, emotional state or similar factors. These two aspects suggest different treatment approaches which can be used separately or together.

Physical Basis

There are terminals called **receptors** at the end of the nerve fibers running through our body. These receptors are located in the skin, muscles and organs. The receptors and nerves which are most often implicated in peripheral neuropathy of the type we are mainly discussing are **sensory** (as opposed to motor or autonomic). These are the ones receiving and transmitting signals of feeling and touch.

Electrical impulses from the sensory receptors are sent through the nerve fibers to the **spinal cord** and then are relayed on to the brain for processing. If the impulses are distorted, magnified or multiplied, pain may be perceived when the impulses reach the brain. These distortions or other changes in impulses may be the result of (a) the **degeneration of the axon** of the nerve cell or of the **nerve cell** itself, thereby changing the conduction properties of the nerve impulses or (b) the **destruction of the myelin sheath** around the nerve, greatly altering the rate and timing of impulse conduction to and from the spinal cord. Either axon or myelin sheath damage can result in motor weakness or abnormal sensation including pain.

The nerve trunks contain both large and small nerve fibers. The **large** fibers carry impulses faster than the small ones and are conduits for unpleasant PN sensations such as **"pins and needles"** and **"tight band"** perceptions as well as **numbness** and **tingling**. (Tingling is an indication of damage or irritation to the nerves in the area affected; numbness suggests the nerve is dead or severed.) **Small** nerve fibers transmit **pain signals** as well as sensations of **hot** and **cold**. Damage to small fibers results in **burning** and **aching sensations** which are usually persistent.

Neurotransmitters are chemical substances located in each nerve cell. They are the messengers which relay nerve impulses to the brain. Neurotransmitters will be dealt with in more depth later but suffice it to say here that they can act either as pain killers or pain generators.

The brain produces neurotransmitters itself called **endorphins** which can have a powerful effect in reducing pain. The effect is much the same as if a person were taking heroin or morphine. (Joggers and runners are familiar with this endorphin effect, sometimes called "runners' high." Every now and then, in the good old days when I was able to jog, I would get a wonderful euphoric feeling after running 30 or 40 minutes. The endorphins would kick in and make me feel like I could run forever-or at least another half mile.)

An interesting theory has recently been advanced concerning the physical basis of neuropathic pain. According to this, an excessive level of proteins called **cytokines**, manufactured by the immune system to promote healing, is a causative factor. It is believed that the specific cytokine culprit is **Interleukin-6**. This protein is expressed by neurons in the spinal cord after injuries and may not only help promote healing but also cause the spinal cord to generate neuropathic pain sensations in the process. Research indicates cytokines may also inhibit **nerve regeneration**.

Support for this theory is thought to lie in the fact that the level of these cytokines in the body appears to peak when perceptions of pain peak. This observation, if it proves true and meaningful, in turn could lead to a new class of pain killers based on drugs that block the action of Interleukin-6.

Psychological Basis

According to a theory called "**gate control**," nerve impulses are regulated at a theoretical "gate" in the spinal cord which transmits or blocks pain signals at the brain's discretion. The Pain Center of Scripps Memorial Hospitals has published a paper, "You and Pain," which refers to an earlier study (by Drs. Melzack and Wall in 1965) claiming that positive emotions such as joy and a sense of well-being tend to close the gate and inhibit pain sensations. Negative emotions such as fear and anxiety open it and allow the transmission of these sensations.

Some researchers, expressing a slightly different view of pain generation, say that nerve impulses giving rise to the kind of **chronic pain** experienced by many PNers actually travel a different pathway than does **acute pain**, and that these impulses pass through the area of the brain (the "thalamus") where emotions (and emotional problems, such as depression) are controlled. They argue that this factor suggests a direct relationship between chronic pain and emotions.

It is also thought there may be a relationship between a person's psychological state and the *intensity* of the pain experience. According to this analysis, **stress**, **depression**, or **anxiety** can all increase the intensity of pain. Consequently, it is contended that procedures which reduce these factors will tend to lessen pain intensity.

In summary, many researchers believe pain is the result of a number of interwoven physical and psychological factors and that it has both a subjective, mental as well as an objective, physical basis.

Chapter 3

Pain Medications

Introduction

Although there is presently no true *cure* for PN, there are particular neuropathies which can be successfully **treated** by dealing with their **underlying causes**. Treatment as used here means attempting to restore the patient to some degree of normalcy, to bring the affected PNer back to where (or as close as possible to where) he or she was before the onset of the disorder. These neuropathies include:

- diabetic neuropathy, which as noted in Chapter 8 can be controlled most effectively by lowering blood sugar levels;
- neuropathies induced by vitamin deficiencies, toxins and certain drugs, corrected by supplementing the deficiency (covered in Chapter 6) or by removing the causative agent;

- autoimmune and inflammatory neuropathies treated by plasmapheresis, IVIg, or immunosuppressive medications, discussed in Chapter 4;
- certain motor neuropathies managed by physical and psychotherapies covered in Chapter 5 or orthopedic interventions mentioned in Chapter 9;
- certain autonomic neuropathies treated symptomatically, such as with medications (**metoclopramide**, for example) which increase gastric emptying, and drugs to maintain standing blood pressure, treat sexual dysfunction, aid in emptying the bladder (such as **bethanechol**) and treat diarrhea or constipation; and
- paraneoplastic—tumor-related—neuropathies, mentioned in a footnote in the previous chapter, treated by eliminating the tumor.

Unfortunately, though, most PNers, including many having neuropathies of the types just listed, must also deal with associated pain. This chapter deals mainly with medication therapies designed to alleviate **neuropathic pain**.

General

Many pain killers are either **over-the-counter analgesics** such as aspirin and acetaminophen (Tylenol), or **opioids** like morphine or codeine. Unfortunately, the former generally are considered either too weak or not well targeted to PN pain. The latter are thought by some practitioners to have too many undesirable side effects. Additionally, although opioids appear useful in some cases, they are often considered ineffective with neuropathic pain.

A number of other medications originally approved by the FDA for non-PN purposes are currently being used to treat PN pain. Doctors have long been able to properly prescribe these drugs for "off-label" (non-FDA approved) applications. It has only been recently, however, that pharmaceutical companies have been allowed to actively advertise and promote these uses.

Below is a survey of some of the more commonly prescribed **non-opioid medications** for neuropathic pain. The emphasis here is on the kind of pain principally addressed, the classification of the drug, various side effects (not intended to be exhaustive) and typical dosages being used. I have included some but not extensive detail concerning reported mechanisms of action since they sometimes are either debatable or are just too complex for purposes of this book. (For instance, is knowing that a particular drug results in an inhibition of prostaglandin biosynthesis really meaningful or helpful to most of us PNers?)

The discussion which follows also is obviously not meant to suggest any particular medication for anyone. Your attending physician needs to consider in detail with you the appropriateness and use of any specific drug, including limitations, contraindications and drug interactions. The discussion *is* meant, though, to prod you and your doctor into *thinking* about some of these medications based on information that is available. In this arena it's a "given" that what works for one may not work for someone else. It oftentimes is a matter of trial and error until the right drug or combination of drugs is found.

By the way, in looking at PNer comments with respect to various drugs you may be surprised to see how many are on a combination of different medications and nutrients. If such a PNer suddenly notices an improvement in symptoms it may be difficult to correctly identify which particular substance in the "cocktail" is doing the job.

If you are presently on a medical regimen that's not working for you and it's been given enough time to do so, or if you're having difficulty with side effects, you should ask your physician about trying a different medication. Remember, **you** are the patient and even though you can't self-prescribe, you have the right to be the final arbiter of your own situation. Most doctors understand this. (But don't be intimidated if yours doesn't! If this approach happens to bother him or her, consider changing something more than your medication.)

On the subject of doctors, there are good arguments for initially taking your PN symptoms to a competent **neurologist**—a medical doctor who specializes in the evaluation and treatment of nerve disorders. Such a specialist is equipped by training and background to assess your condition. (Even here it is wise to determine in advance that the particular neurologist you are considering is experienced in dealing with peripheral neuropathy!) Moreover, a neurologist is much more likely than most practitioners to fearlessly prescribe a large enough dosage of the chosen medication, based on specialized knowledge, to achieve the desired result. Many PNers who have gone through multiple medical professionals, spending much time and much money in the process, will loudly attest to all of this!

Non-Opioid Drugs

Bearing in mind that categorization is a bit subjective and that the lines sometimes blur, the following discusses which drugs seem to be prescribed most often by doctors for the particular types of neuropathic pains listed. Drs. Catherine Willner and Phillip A. Low in their study, "Pharmacologic Approaches to Neuropathic Pain" (included in the treatise, *Peripheral Neuropathy,* Dyck & Thomas, W. B. Saunders, 1993), suggested the following guidelines a physician might use in making a particular choice:

> "The choice of a specific drug used in the treatment of neuropathic pain in a particular patient is preceded by a comprehensive assessment of the type (s) of pain experienced by the patient, the impact of the pain on the patient's functioning, the underlying pathophysiologic mechanisms, and the limiting medical conditions or contraindications. Knowledge of the natural course of the painful neuropathy is also relevant."

Here then are the non-opioid drugs most commonly being used to deal with pain:

1. **for burning pains**:
    (a) all of the so-called tricyclic antidepressants including Elavil (amitriptyline)[1] (this one particularly where sleep disorders are a problem); Norpramin (desipramine); Pamelor (nortriptyline); and Tofranil (imipramine)
    (b) Mexitil (mexiletine hydrochloride)
    (c) Neurontin (gabapentin)
    (d) Ultram (tramadol)

2. **for shooting, stabbing, "electric shock" pains**
    (a) Dilantin (phenytoin)
    (b) Klonopin (clonazepan)
    (c) Neurontin (gabapentin)
    (d) Tegretol (carbamazepine)

3. **for aching, persistent pains**
    (a) Catapres (clonidine)
    (b) Klonopin (clonazepan)
    (c) Lioresal (baclofen) (particularly when accompanied by spasms and cramping)
    (d) Neurontin (gabapentin)

None of these drugs is likely to eliminate our neuropathic pains totally nor restore us to our pre-PN condition completely. What we should be seeking with our

---

[1] Throughout I've adopted the practice of giving the trade name first with the generic name in parentheses since with a few exceptions (baclofen instead of Lioresal, mexiletine instead of Mexitil, clonidine instead of Catapres) most people generally refer to these drugs by their trade names.

doctor is the single medication or combination which will give us the **most relief** with the **fewest adverse side effects**.[2]

1. *Elavil (amitriptyline); Norpramin (desipramine); Pamelor (nortriptyline); Tofranil (imipramine)*

These drugs are **antidepressants** and are further classified as **tricyclics** (a term referring to their chemical structures). They have long been considered effective in treating PN pain, particularly of the burning type. (Interestingly, patients who benefit from these drugs report pain relief before any uplift in mood.) Studies of patients with diabetic neuropathy reportedly suggest that 60% of patients get 50% or more pain relief from tricyclic antidepressants.[3]

The tricyclics appear to act in a common manner. There are microscopic gaps between nerve cells called

---

[2] A neurologist told me he regards success as a 50% reduction in a patient's pain level. He increases whatever medication is being used, from a low start point gradually until the 50% reduction is reached or until the patient cannot tolerate the side effects of the medication.

[3] One needs to be careful in not relying too much on conclusions of pain relief from reported studies. Various biases can creep in even where "objective" measuring techniques and rigorous protocols are being used. Obviously studies which are not even randomized or placebo-controlled are especially suspect. After looking at hundreds of studies for this book my conclusion is that the more recent the study the greater is the credibility that probably can be attached to it. This is undoubtedly because investigators have been steadily improving their techniques and tightening their analytical methods over the years.

synapses. For a nerve impulse to travel from one nerve cell to another, the sending cell releases a tiny amount of a chemical called a neurotransmitter. This chemical carries the nerve impulses across the synapses. Depression is strongly associated with abnormally low levels of these neurotransmitters. Tricyclic antidepressants increase their levels and the duration of their action by a process called "**reuptake inhibition**." This inhibitory action elevates the brain's threshold to pain.

Side effects of the tricyclics include possible blurred vision, dizziness, dry mouth, constipation, weight gain and occasionally excessive perspiration. Patients may also experience palpitations and urinary retention. Practitioners emphasize that patients should be told to stop taking their medication if these problems occur. (Dr. Jane E. Mahoney, University of Wisconsin School of Medicine, in a letter to *The New England Journal of Medicine* [Sept. 21, 1995], suggested that Elavil should be avoided in elderly diabetic patients when other treatment options are available. Her reasoning was that it can exacerbate problems such as the constipation and urinary retention to which older people with diabetes are often prone.)

Elavil, being the most sedating of the four drugs, is believed particularly helpful when given at night to patients having **sleep problems** secondary to their pain. Sometimes another tricyclic antidepressant is prescribed for daytime use in combination with Elavil at night. (Of the four tricyclics mentioned, Norpramin is considered the least sedating.)

Dosages are tailored to the patient's needs. The amount required to provide pain relief is generally lower than the dosage required to treat depression. Sometimes physicians treating PN will start with 10 mg to 25 mg daily for **Elavil** and **Pamelor** and 100 mg for **Norpramin** and **Tofranil**. If there is no response after 2 weeks, dosages are often "titrated" (medicalese for increased) in 25 mg increments every 2–3 weeks until pain relief or undesirable side effects are experienced. Rarely is it thought necessary to go over 150 mg per day for Elavil and Pamelor, or 300 mg daily for Norpramin and Tofranil. Elderly persons and patients with advanced liver disease are usually limited to lower doses.

With any antidepressant it's considered especially important that the patient be on the medication long enough to give the drug a chance to work. Some practitioners advise their patients to wait at least several weeks before giving up.

When the tricyclic antidepressants are not well tolerated there are several *non-tricyclic* antidepressants sometimes prescribed for PN patients. Often they are used in combination with other medications such as Neurontin. These non-tricyclics are strong **serotonin reuptake inhibitors**—a class of antidepressants which promotes the transmission of nerve impulses using the neurotransmitter serotonin. Included are **Effexor (venlafaxine)**, **Paxil (paroxetine hydrochloride)**, **Prozac (fluoxetine)** and **Zoloft (sertraline)**. In the past they have been aimed more at counteracting depression than for pain relief.

Incidentally, I thought the following comment from

Dr. Steven King, actively involved in psychopharmacology work at the University of Chicago, was interesting in choosing among the tricyclic antidepressants:

"The literature shows nortriptyline [Pamelor] is just as effective as amitriptyline [Elavil]. . . . The only advantage of amitriptyline is the added sedation since many pain patients have difficulty sleeping. My rule of thumb is if sleeping is a major problem and there are no contraindications to amitriptyline, I'll start with it. If sleeping isn't a problem, I'll try desipramine [Norpramin]. I go with it instead of nortriptyline because it's much less expensive and works as well with regard to analgesia."

Following are patient comments on the principal drugs covered in this sub-section. It should be kept in mind that none of these, and none of the patient comments which appear elsewhere in this book, can be relied upon as medical opinions or treatment guides. You should always consult your doctor with regard to any particular medication or other therapy.

[comments re Elavil are not to be considered medical opinions and should not be relied upon as such—always consult your doctor:

(1) I've been taking Ultram for three years. I also take 600mg Tegretol and 1800 mg Neurontin. Help!!!!!!! I still have severe pain during the day. At night, around 6:00 p.m., when I take the 150 mg **Elavil** with 200mg Tegretol and 600mg Neurontin I'm out like a light in 1hr. 45min. It doesn't matter what I'm doing, I'm going out. I sleep pain free till 5:00 a.m. It is good sleep too. Robin

(2) I take 200mg **Elavil**. I had to take off work to go from 25mg to 200mg. I had to put in for medical retirement so you can see I can't work any more. It helps with the pain or I should say the constant pain isn't so bad but the stabbing pain still comes. Mostly it helps to sleep at nite. My head and body shake and I have it in my hands, arms, feet and legs. I wish you good luck. Christy

(3) **Elavil,** Elavil, Elavil. I take 100mg and boy! what a difference in the pain. Darvocet for when I have extreme pain. But the big difference came around when the dr. started the Elavil, also called amitriptyline. It can be taken in combination with other things. It was like a miracle when it kicked in. The dr. did a blood test to make sure enough was getting in my system to make the difference. It also makes one feel good as it is an antidepressant. But the real good thing is the pain relief. Joan

(4) I am on Serzone which is a form of an antidepressant and MS Contin, morphine. I have tried others also but nothing really helps. I was on **Elavil** but that caused a big weight gain. Since I stopped it I have lost 62 pounds!!!! Lee

(5) I've been taking 10 mg of **Elavil** per day for the past week, and I am completely amazed at the result. For the first time in years I am without the regular aching burning pain in my hands and feet. I never would have expected anything to be this effective. I literally stop what I'm doing several times a day to note that I am not feeling pain. When I think back on what I put up with for all those years, I am truly sorry I didn't find out about this sooner. Anon

(6) My peripheral neuropathy (a sensory neuropathy) has been treated (managed) on a long term basis (20 years) quite successfully. . . . My neurologist is successfully treating my condition with amitriptyline HCL [**Elavil**]. Once an appropriate dose was found (it varies from person to person) my pain has been almost completely managed so I have hardly

any restrictions on activities I can participate in. One very important thing about taking this prescription drug—amitriptyline HCL—is that the dosage must be ramped up very slowly. Each time that the dosage is increased you feel extremely lethargic and sleepy. But after a few days at a given dosage this effect completely disappears and, if needed, another increase in dosage can then be tried. Also, if you stop taking it—the drug remains in your body for many weeks. My peripheral neuropathy (sensory neuropathy) is currently being successfully managed by 150mg of amitriphyline HCL per day taken at night. An unusual effect that I discovered is that my general attitude can cause the return of my symptoms. An example of this is when my cat died. I was greatly emotionally affected and my symptoms returned. After a period of time my mood returned to normal and my symptoms went into general remission again. I have experienced similar episodes similar to this 2 or 3 more times over several years. Lane

(7) I take **Elavil** for the burning. When it starts up again in a more intense way I ask the dr. to increase the dose of the Elavil because I know it works for me. Dr. said one becomes tolerant to doses eventually and they have to be increased. I take 60 mg. at night now. Started with 25. Can go up to 150 with no problem, she says, so I have a way to go. Sometimes increasing by only 10 mg at a time helps make the difference. Joan

(8) I am a non insulin type II diabetic, work full time at a large university. I have found a cadre of medications that make work possible but my physician will treat the pain for a while but then refuses to refill with strong enough dosages to control pain . . . as if my problem were like a cold that will get better. I am in pain, getting depressed and am desperate. I take glucophage, Mexitil, Surmontil and Ultram. Tried amitriptyline [**Elavil**] what a horror. Help! ML

(9) If it's neuropathy, something that may help (though you probably need a visit with a neurologist to confirm) is small doses of tricyclic antidepressants, such as nortriptyline or amitriptyline [**Elavil**]. Women can usually start with only 10 mg a day. If the pain makes it hard to sleep, I suggest trying the amitriptyline about an hour before bedtime because it's pretty sedating. There are some unpleasant side effects, but it often helps put the pain on a back burner (though it doesn't eliminate it completely). Also, my personal experience is that I need higher and higher doses to combat the pain. The drugs are a stopgap measure, but, for me anyway, they help a lot. Paula

10) I am a 28 year old female that was diagnosed with PN about 2 1/2 years ago. I went to England and Ireland for vacation in April of 96. It was there that I noticed a neuralgia type pain in my upper back. I ignored it as stress from traveling and went on as usual. On my return . . . about 2 weeks later . . . I started getting this burning sensation in my legs and arms. I was VERY scared! At first I thought it might be MS and was horrified. I went to several doctors that were completely clueless and I usually came home crying due to my pain and frustration. Finally I went to a neurologist who gave me some simple tests and told me that I had PN. He said he had no idea as to why I had it but one of his suggestions was that I had a flu/cold that remained in my nervous system. He prescribed **Elavil** which was a dream come true! Other then the slight weight gain and nighttime drowsiness; the pain went away! I was on it for a year and the only thing I noticed from the PN was a slight weakness in my arms and right leg. Just for the record I would like to note that I was in a horrible relationship at the time and was under terrible stress. Whether this had anything to do with it . . . I will never know. I met the man of my dreams about a year after and got married. At which time I decided to go off Elavil

AND start multi-vitamins to see if pain would return. I was a bit nervous but after a month of being Elavil free I had no pain whatsoever and no weakness for over a year now. I feel great and I truly believe the PN is gone! I would only have to say that once in a blue moon do I get a sort of pin prick say in my arm. I hope this is an inspiration to anyone with PN. I know what you are going through. JC]

[comments re Norpramin are not to be considered medical opinions and should not be relied upon as such—always consult your doctor:

(1) For the burning pain, I also take desipramine [**Norpramin**], an anti-depressant that does not put me to sleep like Elavil does. In fact, I take it in the a.m. because I was not sleeping well when taking it before bedtime. As has been written time and again, it's all trial and error re relief and so far there is no cure. Marjorie

(2) After the results of the tests came back, I too have idiopathic neuropathy. He said he could only relieve my discomfort and put me on desipramine [**Norpramin**]. It is an antidepressant (I am not depressed) used to relieve the uncomfortable feeling in my feet. I have been on it for three weeks and am able to walk farther than before the drug. I also am able to sleep better. However I do feel at times that the pain is spreading. I too am not going to give up. Eldon]

[comments re Pamelor are not to be considered medical opinions and should not be relied upon as such—always consult your doctor:

(1) I have been on Elavil for just about 6 months. I am now taking 125 mg a day. I had been on **Pamelor** for a couple of months, but I get much more relief from the Elavil. My neurologist gives me a prescription for 125 mg a day, but has them dispensed in 25 mg doses so I can adjust as I feel

the need, up or down. I am the most comfortable on125, but I really like the feeling that I can change as my body needs more or less help. Ginny

(2) Went Friday to the neurologist and he put me on **Pamelor** to help me sleep without the itching. Says that 2400mg/day of Neurontin is about at the top of what he will prescribe, and to try the Pamelor for a while. Diana

(3) Nortriptyline [**Pamelor**] is an antidepressant, but it has the side effect of causing weight gain through an increase in appetite. It still does provide the effect of pain control, (as you can get with amitriptyline) but you may still have the effect of weight gain. These drugs are widely known for pain relief but there is more to them . . . I took it for a period of time to increase appetite and gain weight. Darcy

(4) When I was first diagnosed with PN I was prescribed nortriptyline by my neurologist, as **Pamelor.** It is one of several tricyclic anti-depressants (Elavil and Desipramine are a couple of the others) which work against PN pain. I was told that they did not know WHY it worked, but that it did. And it worked for me for several years. However, one nasty side effect was a very dry mouth. Despite a stash of Tic-Tacs in every pocket and purse, I really suffered. Sometimes I awoke in the a.m. with the insides of my throat actually stuck together. Finally, my neurologist switched me to Neurontin, and I have been happier, and without the dry mouth. With the addition of an additional 800mg Motrin I can usually make it through the night. Rose Anna]

[comments re Tofranil are not to be considered medical opinions and should not be relied upon as such—always consult your doctor:

(1) Two years ago, I was diagnosed with PN after having a EMG and nerve conduction tests. The neurologist started me on imipramine [**Tofranil**] which relieved the leg pain enough that I could go to work. Robert

(2) I have been diagnosed with peripheral neuropathy. It has affected my feet, legs, back and arms. The pain and the burning is sometimes unbearable. The neurologist that examined me said I also have fibromyalgia and he put me on 75 mgs of imipramine [**Tofranil**] a day. It has relieved the pain, depression and burning. Anon

(3) I went to a new neuro yesterday who specializes in PN. He had some very new and exciting news for me. First of all my EMG was normal-the other neuro said it showed severe PN. He said that the fibers within the nerve itself are the ones that are affected in my PN. He asked about symptoms and I told him that I no longer had any burning, pain or pins and needles. He tested my legs (my left always being the worst) and I found I now have feeling in my thigh, which was not there two months ago. He said that whatever I am doing it is working. I am on 50 mgs of imipramine [**Tofranil**] per day. The first neuro said that this would help the nerves to relax and heal themselves. This neuro agreed and said to continue taking it as it is doing the job. He said that sometimes we can heal our own bodies. One thing this has shown me is that everyone should definitely get at least two opinions! I had to share this with everyone because I believe there is always hope. I also believe that everyone must concentrate on overcoming the disease not the disease overcoming us. I read once, "What you think, you are." Anon

(4) The neurologist that I went to put me on 75 mgs of imipramine [**Tofranil**] and told me that it should take about three months for my nerves to start to heal. I went for the EMG and he said I have severe PN and nothing could be done for the damage that has already occurred. But he did say that if I stay on the imipramine that the nerves will start to heal. He wants me back in 6 mos. I am still not sure of this but the imipramine has helped with the pain. I have had other sensations in other areas since I

have begun with this medication. I have been told that the
pain is much worse when your nerves start to heal.]

2. Mexitil (mexiletine hydrochloride)

Mexitil is a relatively new drug which has been used
mainly to treat heart problems. Recently it has shown
promise in the treatment of neuropathic pain, particularly of the burning type. It is a **sodium channel
blocker** and an **oral analog** of **lidocaine**—a local anesthetic used by dentists. Lidocaine, in fact, is sometimes
used intravenously before Mexitil is prescribed in order
to predict whether Mexitil will be effective.

Mexitil is believed to work by effectively slowing the
rate and intensity of pain impulses entering the body's
"pain gateways" (gate control theory was discussed in the
previous chapter) which lie along the spinal cord at junc-
tions where major peripheral nerve trunks enter.

Results from one placebo-controlled trial for HIV-
related neuropathy indicated that eight out of ten patients experienced 50% pain relief with Mexitil.

Dr. Robert Vander Griend of Gainsville, Florida, reported on another study involving 35 patients with diabetic neuropathy. (The report was published in a July 17,
1997, news release from the American Orthopaedic Foot
and Ankle Society.) One hundred and fifty mg of mexiletine was administered two or three times a day to the
group, the exact amount adjusted on the basis of response to the treatment, for three months. At the end of
that period the dosage was gradually decreased. If pain
returned a patient would be started back at the lowest

effective dose. Thirty-two patients reportedly noticed a reduction in pain, rating their improvement 50% on average. Three suffered nausea and had to stop. According to Dr. Vander Griend, about half the patients showed long lasting improvement even after the medication was discontinued.

In a study reported in the March 1998 issue of *Diabetes Care,* Swedish researchers recruited 126 adults with diabetic neuropathy. One-quarter were given a placebo; the others took mexiletine for three weeks. The mexiletine group reportedly had significantly less pain at night and slept more peacefully than the group taking the placebo, according to the investigators. The people on mexiletine reportedly did experience some slight side effects such as nausea, abdominal pain and diarrhea.

However, Mexitil is generally well tolerated. Possible side effects include stomach upset (which might be reduced by giving the drug with food or antacids) as noted in the Swedish study, dizziness and sedation. One neurologist told me that before starting a patient on Mexitil the physician should rule out any history of heart disease and, in particular, any history of arrhythmia.

Mexitil is usually started at a dosage of 150 mg to 200 mg at bedtime and then increased to the same amount twice a day and then three times a day, balancing pain relief against side effects. Reportedly, it may take several weeks to begin relieving pain.

[comments re Mexitil are not to be considered medical opinions and should not be relied upon as such—always consult your doctor:

(1) I also am new to this site and have had neuropathy for about five years. I have diabetes and this probably is the cause of my disease. I have been given amitriptyline along with Neurontin with little success. I have found a new doctor who took me off the Neurontin and amitriptyline and prescribed **MEXITIL** and that has been fairly successful. I have learned that nothing will take the pain completely away but the MEXITIL has been the best thing I have taken yet and with little side effects. John

(2) I have run the full gauntlet of drugs and have found the only one with manageable side effects (poor coordination and some mental confusion) is **Mexitil**. This is an anti-arrhythmic drug that has lidocaine which is a pain killer commonly use in dentistry. Helps heaps with the pain and tingles to a lesser degree. Like all the drugs it doesn't suit everyone nor eliminate the disease and all it's consequences, but for me it works. Jessie

(3) Ask your doctor to consider treating you with **Mexitil**. This is an oral lidocaine (like the dentist uses to put your teeth asleep); but available in pill form. It is effective in many (but not all) patients with PPN (painful peripheral neuropathy), especially the burning component of this pain. Robert

(4) Some drugs are best for burning pain (antidepressants, for example), others are best for aching and stabbing pain. Nothing will make you like new. I personally have found most relief from an oral version of lidocaine called mexiletine [**Mexitil**] (which was prescribed by an anesthesiologist at a pain management practice). Marjorie

(5) I take mexiletine [**Mexitil**] and have for 6–8 months now with no problems at all. I started out @ 240 MGs twice a day along with the other pain meds: Oxycotin 10MGs TID and Visteril 25MGs and Visteril ES for break through

pain. No more than 8 a day. I can get through my day not pain free but some what comfortable. As I said I have had NO problems with this drug @ all. I think it is great. Hang in there and have a great, less pain filled day. Good luck Dale

(6) I just started taking mexiletine [**Mexitil**], but has caused headaches and sore throat. Is this normal and will side effects diminish over time? I discontinued use for now, but I am considering trying again. I had a bad reaction from Neurontin at first, but after continued use the side effects diminished. Leonard

(7) Mexitilene [**Mexitil**] helps with the burning and pain. I've been taking it for about 4 months now. I take 3 capsules 3x daily along with 5 mg. of Methadone. I take 150 mg. elavil at night for sleep. I am the most PAINFREE I have been in 3 yrs. I still have bad days but they are becoming less frequent. I still have daily pain, it's just tolerable now. Robin]

3. Neurontin (gabapentin)

Neurontin is an **anticonvulsant** originally developed to control **epileptic seizures**. It is now the first line agent on many lists of pharmaceuticals used for neuropathic pain of various types. There are a number of clinical and anecdotal reports as to its efficacy.

In late 1998 the *Journal of the American Medical Association* (*JAMA*) reported a national multi-center study of 165 patients with diabetic peripheral neuropathy who had received Neurontin over an eight-week period. The patients enrolled had a one- to five-year history of neuropathic pain. Results indicated that approximately 60%

taking the drug had at least moderate improvements in their PN pain compared to only 33% who were given placebos.[4] In addition, the medication proved to be well-tolerated; two-thirds of the Neurontin patients were able to take the highest dosage tested (3600 mg daily) though many were apparently receiving benefits at lower levels.

Neurontin is often times considered helpful in suppressing burning pains as well as those of the shooting and persistently aching types. (As you will see from the following comments of users, though, as well as from the above-mentioned survey, it certainly doesn't help everyone. But then no other drug does either.)

The mechanism of action has not been clearly established, according to the manufacturer. However, all anticonvulsant drugs, used mainly to quiet excessive brain discharges accompanying epileptic seizures, may also quiet the pain distress signals associated with peripheral neuropathy. One way they may do so is by enhancing the effects of **GABA**, an inhibitory neurotransmitter which helps prevent our nerve cells from "firing too fast."

Side effects of Neurontin appear to be limited mainly to drowsiness, dizziness or upset stomach. In general, it is believed to be better tolerated than most drugs used to treat neuropathic pain.

Some physicians start the dosage at 300 mg a day,

---

[4] The "placebo effect" is a well documented phenomenon. Statistics indicate that on average one-third of subjects in a clinical trial will report improvement simply from a sugar pill or other placebo. To demonstrate that a treatment is effective one must show it performs significantly better in the treated group than in the control or placebo group.

titrated up to 2400 mg or even 3600 mg a day in three doses. (Each dose is said to be effective for four to five hours.) Many doctors feel most patients begin to experience pain relief at a daily dose of 900–1200 mg. A number of practitioners emphasize titration should be done slowly and carefully to find the minimum level at which the drug is effective.

There are reports from some patients that Neurontin works somewhat like aspirin in that it provides relief even when taken sporadically—on an "as needed" basis. Anyone using this medication, however, should consult with his or her physician before relying on that approach.

[comments re Neurontin are not to be considered medical opinions and should not be relied upon as such—always consult your doctor:

(1) The best thing I've found for the burning, stabbing and electrical feeling that I get has been **Neurontin**. I've tried all of the other anti-depressant type drugs and this one is great. It comes in 300mg capsules and I take 1800mg a day. Tim

(2) Just wanted to jump on the bandwagon of relief and tell y'all I had a PAIN FREE 7 hours today!!! What a treat! I just couldn't believe it, first in weeks. My doc upped my **Neurontin** to 300 mgs 4x daily and the Klonopin to daytime use. Really seemed to do the trick. Laura

(3) Thought I was only person in the world with something called peripheral neuropathy! I'm 3 years new to the condition and taking **Neurontin** with only little effect. Anne

(4) I have been taking **Neurontin** for three years for PN. I take 2400 mg a day to control the burning pain in my legs, arms, hands and face. My doctors have explained the orig-

inal purpose of Neurontin was to prevent seizures for people who suffer from epilepsy. In PN cases it blocks the pain signals in the brain. It usually is accompanied with another pain drug. For me at this high dose, I get about 50% relief. Side effects include a feeling of pressure on your head, similar to the feeling of having a hat on when you don't, some dizziness, mouth dryness, and short term memory loss. They say these side effects gradually go away, so far they haven't for me. Neurontin works real good when most of your pain is the burning type, some doctors use Tegretol, however the side effects are more severe. If you can tolerate the side effects I highly recommend Neurontin for controlling PN pain. Anon

(5) I've been on **Neurontin** about 3 months—2700 mg day. Seemed to help at first, but now I don't think so. The side effects I've noticed are that my words seem to get jumbled up sometimes when I talk. I've also noticed what I've called a bad headache starting at the nape of my neck and coming up the back of my head and over the top. Kenneth

(6) I take **Neurontin** and have only had a problem with short term memory so far. I started out at 100mg 3 times a day and have just moved to 200mg 3 times a day. I know that this is one of the drugs that we get used to, so I am increasing my dosage slowly to get all I can out of it before I wear it out. Neurontin alone is not enough for me, I also take Oxycontin, Ultram, Prozac. I have Vicodin available for when I get pain spikes. I asked my Pain Dr. for OxyIR and he said that due to the large dose of Oxycontin that he didn't think it advisable at this time. Anon

(7) I had to quit **Neurontin** after about a year because of this same problem [blurred vision]. Although it helped a lot with pain at first, it seemed to lose its effectiveness with time. It also caused me mental slowness and memory problems. On a recent test in Oregon it only worked for 40% of

PN patients. I now take 2 Vicodins in the evening 4 hrs apart and 10 mg Elavil at bedtime. Good luck, Bill.

(8) I have been taking **Neurontin** now for a few months and am up to 2700–3600 mg a day as needed. I do not notice any side effects and it does help the pain—I just recently increased the dosage about 2 weeks ago—It was at 2400 mg a day and didn't seem to be working good enough and the neurologist said sometimes a little more will help a lot. . . . So as needed I can up it to 3600 a day. . . . Seems to be working. . . . She said that some can tolerate it very well. It has to do with how your body metabolizes it. It is also suppose to be good if you are taking many different meds, which I am. Margot

(9) I take 2400mg of **Neurontin** per day and it has helped me SO much. I don't have a lot of pain at this time but do have itching in my feet and a heavy, aching numbness in my arms and hands which is quite uncomfortable. Neurontin does help with those symptoms. I have had these symptoms progress very quickly and know that without Neurontin I would be unable to function. Some haven't had as much success as I have had with the drug, but I would say it has helped the majority who have taken it. Give it a chance and do not be afraid to ask the Dr to up the script if the lower dosages don't seem to help. The most often occurring side effect (from the pharm paper which comes on the bottle—ask the pharmacist for one to read) is rhinitis—a stuffy nose. I can live with THAT side effect! Good luck, Diana

(10) Add me to the **Neurontin** Appreciation Association. I take 600 3x a day . . . it stopped the "shocks", but still have the burning, cramping, ice cold . . . all the rest. But . . . NO SHOCKS! Funny how it can work so differently for each of us. Carol

(11) Several physicians prescribed Tegretol (anticonvulsant) for pain management before **Neurontin** came along.

Neurontin does not require frequent blood tests, and because Tegretol does require monitoring of blood, that is one advantage Neurontin has over Tegretol. Just like every other med taken for pain relief (e.g. Elavil, Neurontin, Paxil, acetaminophen, ibuprofen) each person responds differently to each med. Many doctors experiment with different combinations of prescribed pills. I am taking Methadone because it was formulated specifically to treat pain. However, many doctors (the majority of docs?) don't want their patients taking narcotics for a variety of reasons. Dennis

(12) Originally I was taking 300mg of **Neurontin** 4 times a day, plus sleeping pills (that I was told was not addictive). The Neurontin caused me to have blurred vision, and loss of memory. When I was finally referred to a neurologist at a major medical center and teaching hospital, my new and competent Dr. (a lady neurologist) immediately started reducing my meds. I now take 300mg Neurontin twice daily, and .5 mg of Klonopin at bedtime (it helps by serving as a sleeping pill) however, it is similar to Neurontin. I have no side effects from any of my Meds now. I also take Prednisone (started one year ago on 50mg daily reducing to 15mg daily now). Just remember each of us is different, and one must experiment (with concurrence of your Dr.) for what works for one will not work for another. God Bless. Hoyt]

4. Ultram (tramadol)

Ultram is an analgesic which has been approved by the FDA for use in the United States only recently. Like the previous drugs just discussed, it is often used to minimize burning type pains.

Ultram is not chemically related to opioids but has a mode of action and produces effects similar to some of them, namely dizziness, nausea and constipation. It also can result in **drug dependence** although withdrawal problems, when present, are not considered to be as severe as those caused by opioids such as codeine.

This drug can slow thinking processes. Physical abilities required for driving and operating machinery are impaired when Ultram is used. It should be strictly avoided where alcohol or opioid abuse might be present.

Dosages generally start at 50 mg to 100 mg every four to six hours, as needed, not exceeding 400 mg a day. It is claimed dose adjustments are not required for elderly patients (at least those under 75) unless they have kidney or liver impairment.

A study at Baylor College of Medicine of 131 patients with diabetic neuropathy (reported in the June 1998 issue of *Neurology*) considered the benefits of Ultram administered at an average dosage level of 210 mg per day. The study was multi-centered, placebo-controlled and double blind (meaning the subjects were placed in two different groups, one receiving the drug and the other a placebo with no one, including the researchers, knowing which was which until the conclusion of the study). The researchers concluded that Ultram was "significantly more effective" than placebo for treating neuropathic pain.

[comments re Ultram are not to be considered medical opinions and should not be relied upon as such—always consult your doctor:

(1) I too have tried Dilantin, and Neurontin without pain relief, but received other undesirable side effects. . . . **Ultram** is the only medication I've found that takes the edge

off burning pain and tingling, and for me . . . no unwanted side effects. Woody

(2) I take Neurontin, 2100mg a day, spaced out in 3 doses. I have had NO side effects to this, so I'm very happy. I also take Paxil, which is another antidepressant, but a much newer one, and that also gives me no side effects. When I'm in a lot of pain, I take 100mg **Ultram**. Jenny

(3) I have tried many different drugs, Neurontin, Tegretol, Naprelan, Trentlal, Dilantin. All had potentially serious side effects, and did nothing to relieve the pain. The only thing that has helped me is **Ultram**. I have been taking it for about a year now, and it seems to help. I haven't had any problems with it so far. Kathleen

(4) He also prescribed tramadol (**Ultram**) for neuropathy pain . . . a low but steady dosage of 50mg three times a day after a slow buildup from smaller dosages. I had previously tried both Neurontin and nortriptyline without success. The tramadol is more effective; but certainly not complete relief. I was advised NOT to increase the dosage because of a small risk of a seizure, which is not something I need. Ray

(5) I've been taking **Ultram** for about a year now. I take 200mgs 3x a day. It's the first medication that ever gave me any relief from the constant burning and aching in my feet and lower legs. I've had no side effects from it but my neurologist thinks I should taper the dosage off until I'm down to four a day. I also take hydrocodone and Neurontin 3300mgs a day. They just started me on mexiletine a couple of weeks ago. I've had PN for about 5 years now. I just filed for disability about a month ago and of course the paperwork and the questions are just starting. Bob

(6) I also have diabetic neuropathy. I am 33 years old and couldn't stay on my feet for more than ten mins. at a time

until my doctor gave my a prescription for **Ultram**. This stuff actually works without making you feel stupid. Anon

(7) From what I found out the pain is caused from the coating on nerve "tracts" having worn away so that when a signal is sent via this "tract" it just kinda shoots out in all directions as an electrical charge of sorts. To me it feels like someone stuck a fork in my leg. When I take the **Ultram** the feeling is reduced to a small throb. Anon

(8) I've been using **Ultram** for about 3 years, with no ill effects and no addiction. These days, I take 2–3 daily, down from 6–8 a year ago. I feel that it has allowed me to continue to work, whereas the other analgesics I was taking, such as Darvocet, Percocet, Demerol, and Talwin NX (not all at once) made me too dopey or panicky to do my job. Without Ultram, I'd have had to go on disability. It doesn't upset my stomach, though some people report this symptom. So I hope it isn't declared to be addictive. It sure doesn't fit that profile in my case. My GP prescribed 200 per month, but my insurance carrier for some reason will allow the pharmacy to sell me [only] 136. But nowadays that's more than enough, so I'm not fussing. Anon]

5. Dilantin (phenytoin)

Dilantin is an **anticonvulsant** used primarily to address electric shock pains. These are thought to be related to abnormal firing of injured nerve fibers. This drug is sometimes considered for patients who cannot tolerate Neurontin or Tegretol, the latter more often prescribed for this purpose and covered later. Similarly to the other anticonvulsants, Dilantin is believed to act by depressing synaptic transmissions and reducing nerve excitability.

Some of the side effects and considerations which apply to Tegretol apply here. In addition, there are some indications long-term use of Dilantin can itself cause neuropathy.

Dosage is often begun at 100 mg at night and then increased in 100 mg increments until either pain relief is obtained or a total dose of 300 mg to 400 mg is reached (assuming blood tests remain satisfactory).

> *[comments re Dilantin are not to be considered medical opinions and should not be relied upon as such—always consult your doctor:*
>
> (1) Does anyone have any recommendations for my sister? She's had PN 2yrs. . . . Does anyone know of any herbal or RX options? She has already run thru **Dilantin** too and had to stop—potential liver problems. She is so frustrated with the drug thing she is trying to not take anything and see if that works. Linda
>
> (2) Two years ago, I was diagnosed with PN after having a EMG and nerve conduction tests. The neurologist started me on imipramine which relieved the leg pain enough that I could go to work. After a year and a half I decided to have another EMG to see how things had progressed because of increased pain in the legs and some tingling in the feet. The new EMG showed that there was more nerve damage. The neurologist said there was no better medication and that he had done all that he could for me. I talked to my internist who is really up on PN and he immediately started me on Zoloft, which didn't do any good at all. Then I went on **Dilantin**, which gave me relief from the pain but had some weird side effects so now I am on Neurontin 400mg three times a day and have pain relief but also a lower backache. Is there no relief without side effects? Robert

(3) My husband has been talking **Dilantin** for 40+ years. Seizure control is excellent and blood levels of dilantin are always within normal limits. Within the past two years he has developed a progressive peripheral neuropathy in both hands. This has now progressed to muscle wasting. Multiple studies have ruled out most common problems. His neurologist advises this may be the result of long term Dilantin use. Any articles/books available? J

6. Klonopin (clonazepan)

Klonopin is another **anticonvulsant** drug being prescribed for neuropathic pain of the shooting and stabbing type (as well as for aching pains). According to some researchers, this drug is considered more effective than Dilantin or Tegretol for these lancinating pains. (See, for example, the article, "Pharmacologic Approaches to Neuropathic Pain," mentioned above.)

Since Klonopin produces mental depression, patients receiving the drug are ordinarily cautioned against engaging in hazardous occupations requiring alertness, similarly to Dilantin. They should also be warned about the concomitant use of alcohol or other drugs such as barbiturates which slow the brain's processes.

Side effects can include confusion, amnesia and hallucinations. Periodic blood counts and liver function tests are advisable during long-term therapy with Klonopin. Incidentally, sudden cessation of this medication can cause seizures.

The initial dose for adults ordinarily does not exceed 1.5 mg a day divided into three doses. Dosage is usually increased by physicians in increments of 0.5 to 1 mg every three days until the pain is adequately controlled or until side effects preclude any further increase. Maintenance dosage is generally established for each patient selectively depending upon response. Maximum recommended daily dose is 15 mg to 20 mg.

[comments re Klonopin are not to be considered medical opinions and should not be relied upon as such—always consult your doctor:

(1) I've been taking .5 mg of **Klonopin** 3 to 4 times a day. I've been having trouble with my feet freezing all night. He upped my Klonopin to 2.5 mg all at once at bedtime, then increasing it over time. I took it at 5:00 last night instead of bedtime and I don't even remember getting up from the dinner table. At 11:00 my husband woke me from my chair and I went to bed, slept though the night and woke up feeling great. He said I need to only take it once a day at bedtime, that it would hold up through the next day. We'll see. Velda

(2) I've been complaining to doctors about burning feet for 6 years, and the first four years I was told I had plantar fasciitis—one orthopod even wanted to sever my plantar fascia (no thanks!). I agree that you've got to keep searching for ways to relieve the pain. All docs agree THERE IS NO CURE for PN at this time. Maybe the nerve growth factors hold promise for us. I tried to get in on a clinical test but participants must have diabetes, which I do not have. I find the antidepressant desipramine and the anti-convulsant **Klonopin** (generic clonazepan) take the edge off the pain. Larry

(3) Tegretol was one of the first drugs I was given, in fairly low doses for PN in feet and hands and every time I took it I would become viciously ill about four hours later, with vomiting, dry-heaves, could not keep even a tablespoon of water down. Even my own saliva came up! It may have re-

acted with other drugs I take for other problems. I'm glad it worked for you. I am currently taking a low dose of **Klonopin** and have had some success in pain relief at night with no side effects other than sleeping more than normal. Best wishes, BJ

(4) **Klonopin** was the best thing that ever happened to me to control my PN. I have tried every other drug under the sun, and this is by far the best for me. It caused headache and drowsiness at first, but my system seems to have accommodated well. It works so well that I find I don't even have to take it on a daily basis. My dosage is 1mg. at bedtime when needed. Teddie

(5) I have taken **Klonopin** for 5 years, 5mg three times a day. I, too, take Tegretol but my new neurologist wants me to try Neurontin and then switch off of the Tegretol. Meanwhile I really feel spacy and get headaches. I started with 1 for a couple days and built up to 3. Klonopin has been a Godsend to me because I have developed tremors in the hands and muscle twitches. I don't know if any of you have experienced it. I hope not. I had to retire and would love to paint, my hand is so shaky, but the Klonopin does calm it. I need a lot of sleep also. The doc can stick pins all the way to my knee now and I can't feel it. Ray

(6) I have taken **Klonopin** several times for PN. It does help the pain and brings on sleep at night, but I shared your experience. I was so drugged during the day that I could not stay awake. During hard days I am tempted to try a 1/2 dose, but usually resist because my brain is the best thing I have right now and I don't want to be groggy. Tegretol zonked me also. I've heard if you wait the drowsiness goes away. Mary

(7) My husband took this medication [**Klonopin**] for restless leg syndrome. The dosage was very small but he developed a severe reaction to the drug . . . itching all over,

so his doctor discontinued it. He was then put on Tylenol 3 with codeine at bedtime and it works well for restless leg syndrome. Anon]

7. Tegretol (carbamazepine)

This is yet another **anticonvulsant** frequently prescribed for PNers, particularly for "electric shock" or stabbing type pains.

Tegretol reportedly has been used successfully for years. In fact the study previously mentioned, "Pharmacologic Approaches to Neuropathic Pain," cited five clinical trials showing the percentage of patients improved ranged from 77 to 100% with improvements ranked from "moderate" to "marked." However, Tegretol is said to interact with a number of drugs and particular caution is advised when combining it with other medicines.

Serious side effects are said to include the possibility of dangerously low blood cell counts, bone marrow suppression, severe skin reactions and serious liver abnormalities such as hepatitis. Minor side effects include dizziness, nausea, and vomiting.

Physicians often begin dosage at 100 mg to 200 mg at bedtime, titrated upwards every two days or so to a maximum of 1200 mg. They say use should be discontinued at the first sign of any blood count abnormality.

[comments re Tegretol are not to be considered medical opinions and should not be relied upon as such—always consult your doctor:

(1) I have been on **Tegretol** for several years and find that it does help the pain. It worked within a week or so. The

trouble with new meds is, we have such high hopes that they will eliminate the pain, that we don't always notice what they are doing for us. It doesn't take care of all the pain, but how I know it works is, when it wears off, I can tell. Velda

(2) I have had **Tegretol** prescribed for me. Dosage started on 1 tablet (100mg) twice daily. It was raised after one week to 2 tablets twice daily. It is scheduled to go to three and finally four. One tablet seemed to work pretty well. It relieved pain (not numbness) and let me sleep. At the two level, I'm like a Zombie. I have a 'phone appointment with my doctor Monday. I will insist that I not go to the three level and that I cut back to one. Bob

(3) I take 600 mg of it [**Tegretol**] three times a day. I think it's probably one of the things that keeps me from going over the edge. A couple times I've tried to cut back and the pain rears its ugly head and makes me realize that no, I don't want to do that. The dose I take is really a bit over the max dose for a day but my neuro checks my Tegretol level occasionally and does liver enzymes often to see where I am. It does mess with some people and they can't take it. In this class of drugs they usually start you out with Dilantin, milder than Tegretol, then move you up to Tegretol if the Dilantin doesn't work. I went right to the Tegretol since the pain was so bad. I've been on it for about 5 yrs. I also take Baclofen, been on it for about 4 yrs. I know the day will come, probably not too far away, when I have to stop taking them both. I try real hard not to think of that time and take it just one day at a time. Shirley

(4) I've had PN for about 10 yrs, first in feet, now both hands and feet. Tried amitriptyline a few days; zonks me out. Used **Tegretol** for about 2 yrs—works OK but didn't like the side effects. Switched to Neurontin. It works about the same as Tegretol for me. Earl

(5) Went to numerous drs. and was given all kinds of reasons initially but finally was told to go to a neurologist. He is prescribing **Tegretol**. Couldn't take it initially because it made me so groggy. Reduced dosage and now increasing it slowly. My feet still burn like crazy especially at night. Anon

(6) I began taking **Tegretol** after being on Dilantin with no favorable results. After 2 weeks of the Tegretol, I noticed a rash on my arms and legs, and a very lethargic feeling. I went into the ER of my HMO, and they ran some blood tests. It came back that my blood platelet count had dropped from a normal 300,000 to 17,000. I was suffering from internal bleeding. The Tegretol helped the pain, but I wound up being in the hospital for 4 days. My advice is to watch for unpleasant side effects. Earl]

8. Catapres (clonidine)

Catapres is an **antihypertensive** drug used especially in the treatment of *diabetic* polyneuropathic pain as well as for "reflex sympathetic dystrophy" (RSD), a chronic pain syndrome typically resulting from trauma to an arm or leg. Catapres may act in the spinal cord, interfering with the transmission of pain signals to the brain. It is sometimes used as a secondary line of defense when other drugs fail to provide pain relief. Another antihypertensive which has been suggested for neuropathic pain is **Minipress (prazosin).**

A special problem limiting the use of Catapres is a condition called "**orthostatic hypotension.**" A significant number of people who take it are said to experience this. Transient low blood pressure (hypotension) often occurs when a person who has been given Catapres suddenly stands up (orthostatic). The resulting dizziness and a feeling of about to black out are said to be due to insufficient blood flow to the brain. In fact, some patients do faint. Drowsiness is reportedly another adverse side effect at higher dosages. Doctors caution that anybody on Catapres should be aware that the sedative effects may be increased by CNS-depressing drugs such as alcohol and barbiturates and that hypotensive effects may be magnified by opioids.

Catapres is usually initiated at a bedtime dosage of 0.1 mg and gradually increased as the above side effects permit. Ultimate doses most commonly employed by doctors seem to range from 0.2 mg to 0.6 mg per day given in divided amounts. Studies have indicated that 2.4 mg is the maximum effective daily dose, but amounts as high as this are rarely employed.

9. Lioresal (baclofen)

This drug is a **muscle relaxant** and **anti-spasmodic**. It also works directly on nerve pathways and, according to some physicians, relaxes or sedates the central nervous system. **Lioresal** is generally reserved for use in dealing with neuropathic pain until after other medications are tried because of troublesome side effects. These may include drowsiness, dizziness, fatigue, headaches and insomnia. Two other muscle relaxants, **Zanaflex (tizanidine)** and **Soma (carisoprodol)**, are sometimes but less often prescribed for neuropathic pain.

Lioresal therapy is usually started at a low dosage, for example, 10 mg taken initially at bedtime for the first two days. Then usage is typically stepped up in 5 to 10 mg increments given in equally divided doses until pain relief is obtained or until a total daily dosage of 80 mg is reached. If results are not obtained after a reasonable trial period physicians most familiar with the therapy recommend that the withdrawal of medication be done gradually to avoid side effects.

Lioresol is sometimes administered by injection through implantable pumps to patients with severe spasticity who are unresponsive to oral therapy.

[comments re Lioresal and Soma are not to be considered medical opinions and should not be relied upon as such—always consult your doctor:

(1) Jim, good luck with the pump. I have one which delivers baclofen [**Lioresal**], a non-opiate anti-spasticity drug. Works pretty well. Had to be replaced after 3 years when it started OD'ing me—watch for symptoms. Mine is refilled every 2 months (I have a pretty low dosage) with minimal inconvenience. Mobile nurses come to my office or home, whichever I specify. Michael

(2) I have been taking **Soma** 350mgs, four times a day. I feel better than I have felt in years. Finally something that helps neuropathy pain. Barry]

Non-Opioid Drug Costs

1. Costs

It is somewhat difficult to talk meaningfully about costs of these medications because there are so many variables. Most but not all are regularly available in **generic** form (see the parenthetical names above), sometimes at substantially reduced prices from the branded product.[5] Also prices may vary markedly among retailers—even, as I found, among pharmacies owned by the same chain in the same city! Nevertheless I thought some price comparisons among the principal drugs discussed above might be helpful.

The "Typical Daily Dose" in the following table is based on dosages indicated in the preceding discussions and on the "typical doses" set forth in the article, "Medication and Pain Management," by Robert W. Allen, M.D., appearing in the *Chronic Pain Workbook*, New Harbinger Publications, 1996. It should be kept in mind, however, that actual dosages may vary significantly from patient to patient and as prescribed by different doctors.

I am using typical prices quoted by pharmacies where I live for generics, to the extent they are available, instead of the branded product. Neurontin and Ultram are

---

[5] Branded or trade-named products are protected by patents for 24 years. Generic products are chemically equivalent compounds which can only be sold after the branded products have lost their patent protection and have entered the public domain. When the generic manufacturer is finally able to sell its "equivalent" product it must meet certain purity standards of the FDA. The generic must also meet certain standards of "bioavailability," which is the amount of medication which actually enters the patient's circulatory system and becomes available therapeutically. However these bioavailability standards can be below those established for the branded products (perhaps sometimes only having 80% of the branded's bioavailability), meaning the patient may not be receiving the same amount of "useable" medication. In certain special cases where medications are very precisely targeted to a particular disease or disorder in a measured way, such as with respect to seizure control, this variance can be critical. If you are concerned about substituting generic for branded products you should discuss the matter with your doctor.

not available in generic form and the branded prices are used. Dilantin is not available locally in its generic form but I have used a price published by Zenith Laboratories, the manufacturer, for the generic.

You undoubtedly will be paying something more or something less than the prices I show depending on where you live, etc., but these prices should be in the ball park. In any event the main purpose of the analysis is to show the *relative* differences among the various drugs when viewed on a typical daily cost basis.

The drugs are listed in the order discussed above:

Name	Typical Daily Dose	Cost Per Day
1. Elavil	25 – 150 mg	$.09 – .54
2. Norpramin	100 – 200 mg	.46 – .92
3. Pamelor	25 – 150 mg	.28 –1.68
4. Tofranil	100 – 200 mg	.48 – .96
5. Mexitil	450 – 600 mg	1.19 –1.59
6. Neurontin *	900 –1200 mg	3.24 –4.32
7. Ultram *	150 – 300 mg	2.25 –4.50
8. Dilantin	200 – 400 mg	.14 – .28
9. Klonopin	1.5 – 4 mg	1.31 –3.50
10. Tegretol	600 –1200 mg	.63 –1.26
11. Catapres	.2 – .6 mg	.20 – .60
12. Lioresal	20 – 60 mg	.48 –1.44

* Not available in generic

2. Payment Assistance

The Congressional Budget Office estimates that about 19 million elderly people have little or no prescription drug coverage. Moreover, an estimated 43 million younger Americans lack health insurance of any kind. It's the elderly and "economically disadvantaged" (the '90s buzz term for the poor and near-poor), though, who especially feel the pinch of high drug costs—costs that can consume 25% or more of a low income family's entire budget.

Unfortunately, **Medicare** does not, with rare exceptions, cover any part of the cost of prescription medications for those over 65. Although about half of Medicare-covered patients are under employer-sponsored plans for retirees or are HMO members, people in the other half have to go it alone unless they have arranged for private insurance such as AARP's **Medigap** program. Sometimes state-run **Medicaid** programs will help those who can't afford drugs but the qualification standards vary drastically from state to state.

Fortunately, there are special programs offered by drug manufacturers to those who need financial assistance. Some 60 companies extend these "**indigent patient programs**" under which free medications are generally given to anyone who does not have the means to pay. Each drug company has its own criteria. For example, Burroughs-Wellcome, manufacturers of **Imuran** (covered later), stipulates that the patient's gross monthly income *usually* (they grant exceptions) must be less than 200% of federal poverty guidelines. This is significantly more liberal than Medicaid standards.

Drug companies usually require that the attending physician initiate the request for assistance and process the necessary forms. (Don't be shy in asking!) A few, though will welcome calls directly from patients for information. For example, Ciba-Geigy, makers of **Tegretol**, has a "Senior Information Assistant" to work with indi-

viduals: 1-800-257-3273. (I'm not sure whether his title
has to do with his status at Ciba-Geigy or with the people he is supposed to assist! I've been too shy to ask.)

Doctors can obtain information from the **Pharmaceutical Manufacturers Association's** (PMA's) web-
site concerning offerings of various member companies
at: www.phrma.org/patients.

To help simplify the paperwork and streamline the
process for you (and for your doctor) there are organiza-
tions which will help for a nominal fee. Two of these are
"The Medication Advocate Program": 1-941-753-2262 ($5
processing fee for each medication requested) and "The
Medicine Program": 1-573-778-1118 (also charges a $5
processing fee).

Topical Medications

Because most of us don't like to take drugs in the first
place, any pain medication in the form of a lotion, cream
or ointment which can be applied externally deserves
careful consideration. For those who have difficulty tolerating the side effects of the drugs listed above, a **surface
treatment** for neuropathic pain relief may be the best
medication choice in many cases.

The principal topical agent being used is capsaicin, a
medication derived from cayenne/red peppers. The potency of peppers has long been appreciated. The Mayans
burned chili peppers to make stinging smoke screens
and flung pepper-filled gourds at their enemies. More recently pepper has been used in sprays to fend off dogs

and would-be assailants. And just as this is being written, Japanese scientists have found a way to keep crop eating monkeys out of farmers' fields by shooting chili powder into the air, irritating the eyes and noses of the luckless primates!

For neuropathic pain capsaicin is delivered either in the form of cream (trade names **Zostrix**—0.025% capsaicin; **Zostrix H.P.**—0.075%; **Axsain**—0.075%) or lotion (**Capsin**—0.025%). Cayenne powder is also supplied in capsule form which is sometimes used for PN pain.

Capsaicin is not an anesthetic but acts to relieve pain by causing nerve cells in the area where applied to release large amounts of a peptide called "**substance P.**" The depletion of this peptide—a neurotransmitter—from nerve endings means that pain impulses cannot be as readily transmitted to the brain.

These products, which do not require prescriptions, are generally applied three to four times daily to the feet or other affected area. An initial burning sensation is usually experienced during the first several days. Continued applications over several weeks are recommended for full results to be obtained. In fact one practitioner told me that if a patient is not willing to use a capsaicin product at least three times a day for an extended period, the patient should not bother with this therapy.

Research results for capsaicin have been impressive. In a multi-center double-blind study[6] involving 277 pa-

---

[6] In a double-blind study neither the researchers nor the subjects know in which group the subjects and in which group the control or placebo subjects have been placed.

tients with diabetic neuropathy (reported in the February 1992 issue of *Diabetes Care*), half being given .075% capsaicin cream and half a topical placebo, 69.5% percent of the group treated with the capsaicin reported significant pain relief. Meaningful differences in walking, working and sleeping measurements were also reported between the two groups at the end of the study.

In another double-blind study at the University of Vermont College of Medicine (reported in the January 1992 issue of *Diabetes Care*), 22 patients with diabetic neuropathy were tested. Half of the group treated with a .075% capsaicin cream over an eight-week period claimed improved pain control. The investigators reported that the mean pain relief on a "visual analogue scale" was 44.6% for the capsaicin group versus 23.2% for the placebo group.

Recently there have been experiments involving cream preparations with a much greater amount of capsaicin than in products currently being offered—in fact up to 100 times more. In these studies a local anesthetic is first injected at the site of the cream application to lessen the intense burning sensation from the high level of capsaicin. In one study (performed at the Department of Anesthesia, University of California–San Francisco and reported in the March 1998 issue of *Anesthesia and Analgesia)* involving 10 patients, the topical preparation was administered over several weeks. Nine reported substantial pain relief which lasted from one to 18 weeks.

Another topical application used sometimes for neuropathic pain is **EMLA**, a mixture of two local anesthetics,

lidocaine (2.5%) and **prilocaine** (2.5%). When combined in a cream these ingredients are able to numb the skin and offer relief. This medication may be useful if one cannot tolerate the burning action of capsaicin. Reportedly, formulations have also been used containing as much as 9–10% lidocaine and 5% of a NSAID (non-steroidal anti-inflammatory drug) such as **ketoprofen** which has analgesic properties. There are other analgesic cream preparations on the market containing **aspirin**, **acetaminophen** or **ibuprofen**.[7]

[comments re Zostrix et al., are not to be considered medical opinions and should not be relied upon as such—always consult your doctor:

(1) When the burning was really horrible, I used a creme called "**Zostrix**," which really helped as long as I followed the directions exactly. Jenny

(2) Biopsy wasn't that bad. Results were chronic inflammatory axonal polyneuropathy with no regeneration. My antibodies are attacking my nerves and destroying both the myelin sheath and the axon. Some kind of autoimmune thing I got after a virus. Not good news. Took 5 days of IVIg—no improvement as yet but it is still early. Don't be afraid of the biopsy it confirms the diagnosis and the severity and the Dr. can then kind of tell you what your future may bring. Treatment is now to address the symptoms. Changed to Prozac because of it's appetite suppressant features and **Zostrix** to

---

[7] One doctor, who told me he had not had much success with Zostrix for neuropathic pain, prescribes either a compound of lidocaine (2%), bupivacaine (2%) and indomethacin (5%), or a ketamine cream, for use 2 to 4 times daily.

rub on my feet and legs. It can be bought over the counter. It does seem to be helping. Kris

(3) I have found that soaking my feet in cool water before going to bed provides a few hours of relief. Also using Ben-Gay or a cream containing capsaicin 0.025% [**Zostrix**] helps very much at night. Richard

(4) Concerning the pain I am taking ELAVIL but what help me more is . . . Pure cayenne yes. It contain a mole-cule: capsaicin which interfere with the feeling of pain. This is the active ingredient of a topical analgesic cream: **Zostrix**. In Canada I find it at the pharmacy. I take 4 cap-sules a day, each contains 470 mg of cayenne powder. Good luck! Jacques

(5) When I started getting serious foot pain from diabetic PN, I found a message in a diabetic forum recommending taking choline (1200 mg daily) and lecithin (2500 mg). I've been doing so for about 3 years now. It seems to help. Best indication is on days when I forget to take them, the pain is worse. I also rub on **Capsaicin** cream (available OTC in various brands now) 3–4 times a day. If I forget that before I go to bed, nighttime pain is worse, so it also seems to work. Bruce

(6) Count me in as one of the "disappointed" users of **Zostrix**. Even used the stronger formula on "advice of doc-tor." Felt like my feet "were eating chili peppers." Best way I can describe the reaction. But then someone suggested I try "Mineral Ice"—a menthol-type solution. . . . I was quite pleased with the "temporary" relief and (jokingly) the aroma even cleared my sinuses. Saul

(7) I have some new lotion that my daughter sent me. It's called "DEEP TISSUE" by Dr. Richard Schultz. It's winter-green Oil, botanical menthol, **cayenne**, ginger root, ar-nica, calendula, and St. Johns wort flowers. It comes in a little bottle with a dropper. I just got it yesterday, but I'm

almost afraid to use it. It has a warning that says "This product is VERY STRONG (their caps)." [Later follow up comment] Surprisingly enough I think the lotion/potion does bring some relief. I've tried it for two nights now and both times I had a relatively quiet night. I still feel the burning but the intensity is a little less. The first night I used rubber gloves to put it on. It really reeks of camphor! Last night I just used my hands and really rubbed it in. Dotti

(8) I take **cayenne** pepper capsules daily as an antidote to neurological pain. I find that it takes both pain and muscle twitching away from me, particularly in my arms from the elbow down. I take 2 capsules 3 times @ day. Always take the capsule(s) with plenty of water and some food. 'Just taking it by itself will most certainly burn your esophagus! Also, a person may want to try the cayenne in liquid form . . . I sometimes use that. I don't know what I would do without my cayenne pepper capsules. Glenn

(9) Has anyone tried the **cream** or gel with **ibuprofen** in it? I am very impressed with how it helps me. I still use the Voltaren and Norflex; but with the cream, I get added relief. Marcia

(10) I am a Certified Pedorthist which means I work with people having foot problems everyday filling prescriptions for their footwear, making custom supports, etc. Most but not all of the PN cases I see are related to diabetes. Many of the people I see say that they get some relief from an ointment with **capsaicin** in it like "Arthritis Rx". Mike]

Other Non-Opioid Analgesics

As previously mentioned, many **over-the-counter analgesics** such as aspirin and acetaminophen (**Tylenol**), intended for general pain relief, or **NSAIDs** such as ibuprofen (**Advil**; **Motrin**) and naproxen (**Aleve**), used both for pain relief and to reduce inflammation, are thought by many not to be very effective in treating neuropathic pain. Often these will be tried first, however, in order to avoid the sometimes severe side effects of prescription drugs. Even these analgesics, however, can lead to problems, particularly after prolonged use. Possible adverse effects include gastric irritation, bleeding and toxicity to the liver (particularly when alcohol is also being used) and kidneys.

Acetaminophen and NSAIDs are said to primarily act by decreasing the production of substances which make nerve endings transmit "painful" impulses back to the spinal cord and onto the brain centers, somewhat in the same fashion as capsaicin.

There are a few NSAIDs requiring prescriptions which are also sometimes used for neuropathic pain. Included are two special formulations of naproxen, **Naprosyn** and **Anaprox**, and **Indocin** (generic is indomethacin).

[comments re other non-opioid analgesics are not to be considered medical opinions and should not be relied upon as such — always consult your doctor:

(1) I know exactly what your husband is talking about. I have been having problems for a year now and I haven't been able to find a drug that gives me my relief. Staying off my feet and extra strength **Tylenol** are the only things that work for me. My feet are stiff and numb and make walking very difficult. Anon

(2) If your husband can't tolerate aspirin, then Advil, Nuprin, Motrin, Relafen, Aleve, or generic Ibuprofen will

also be bad for him. I'm grateful I can tolerate these, because acetaminophen (**Tylenol**) does nothing for me except as a carrier for codeine etc. Michael

(3) Have had the arm & hand pain for yrs. Neuro did test for carpal tunnel. Do have it, but not unusual with PN. The wrist brace is helpful, but my extremely sensitive skin will not allow. The severity of pain comes & goes for me. I take **Tylenol** when it's really bad & try not to aggravate it by using hands less. You will get used to watching your hands carefully when trying to hold onto anything. Just hang in there. It should get better with braces keeping the median nerve "unsquashed". Cherrille

(4) Since the doc has yet to prescribe meds for me (hopefully this week), I have been living off of **ibuprofen**. I take 3 at a time, but it does ease some of the burning. Arline

(5) I am desperately seeking nutritional supplements which will lessen my neuropathy pain. I have been told by a diabetic education 'expert' that the nerve damage cannot be repaired and I may have to live with this pain. She did say that accupuncture might help. I have had two treatments now with no relief, but am not expecting miracles overnight. I am sick of not sleeping. I work full time, and many many days I have to drag to work. I went to bed at 12:30 a.m. and it is now 2:45 a.m. I have been awake nearly an hour due to pain. I have taken a total of 2400 mg of prescription **ibuprofen** in a few hours time with no relief. I KNOW there is help out there. Please SOMEONE help! God Bless all of you suffering out there! La Neta

(6) I have been treated for PN since July, finding some success with Neurontin but the greatest success has been using **Motrin** (600 mg), a warm whirlpool bath at bed time and a warm cup of sleepy-time tea! I take the Motrin before the bath, soak for nearly an hour, and then drink the tea. Within 15min. I can relax in bed. This has been work-

ing for the last week. Maybe next week it won't but I have been in such great pain I'll try anything. Also, I took myself off my pain med, Ultram, and feel much better! I have also begun taking carnitine, folic acid, B complex and omega oils. I have seen some improvement—I'm not using my walker as much. Good luck—we all need it! Nancy

(7) I'm a male 46 w/ diabetes under control w/1 pill a day. I do suffer quite a bit w/ PN in my feet & down one leg. Most of the time its real bad, but you folks all know what it's like. I haven't been to see my MD in about a year, and she insists that I see her this Fri. Diabetes is not her specialty & she is certainly not a neurologist. I do think she is competent and sincere. I'm going to ask her for something that might help ease the PN pain. The problem is that I don't have a clue what to ask for. (She may not know either) I have been taking **Advil** (which I don't think does anything anymore). Tim

(8) I've just started to have problems with my legs, mostly at night. Usually I get up 3 or 4 times and walk. I OD on **Advil**, but it's not working much anymore. Waiting on my mail-order prescription of Neurontin to come in, probably in some UPS truck somewhere. Marilyn

(9) I am taking naproxen **(Naprosyn)**, and it makes a dramatic difference in the pain and inflammation. I was cross-eyed with pain in my hands and later feet but now the pain is minimal. Also, exercise (walking, swimming, lite aerobics) make my feet and hands hurt while I do it and for awhile after, but then my hands and feet feel much better the next day and the difference in my muscles is definitely worth it. Muscle spasms, numbing, pulses, etc. are dramatically better when I exercise. I also have changed my diet and take gross amounts of vitamin and mineral supplements (per a 'health book' from my dentist/friend) and that has slowed the progression dramatically—unfortunately not stopped it. All of the above has improved how I feel and function. Karen

(10) I am also a new member. I do know that **Naprosyn** almost killed me. I was prescribed Naprosyn and Motrin together for gout (now diagnosed as PN) which caused my stomach to hemorrhage. I also doubt that Naprosyn is a cause of PN. While the MDs have not been able to find the exact cause of my PN, I had the symptoms long before I used Naprosyn, and the VA has added PN to the list of conditions caused by agent orange, which I was exposed to in Vietnam in the late 1960s. Anon

(11) I'm taking Soma 375mg two times a day—this works better for me. I also take Elavil 50 mg. at night and **Naprosyn** 500mg two times a day. It takes edge off for me. I have had PN for nine years now. Barry

(12) **Indocin** is more of an anti-inflammatory drug as opposed to pain. I guess you could equate the joint aches with pain, but it isn't really the same as taking something like Percocet or Vicodin. From experience I can tell you to be sure to eat before taking the Indocin. Most of my docs have gone to the 75mg (1 pill/day) Indocin. As long as I don't take it on an empty stomach, the side effects are minimal. David]

Ket (ketamine) is another prescription non-opioid sometimes used for neuropathic pain. It's called a **"dissociative"** drug, meaning that it feels to the person taking it as if the mind is separated from the body. Its chemical structure is related to the illicit drug PCP or "angel dust," and like that substance, Ket can cause hallucinations. Therapeutically, Ket seems to be a quick acting, powerful analgesic when used in smaller doses. It **blocks nerve paths** without depressing respiratory and circulatory functions as do most of the opioids which follow. Studies done using Ket on neuropathic rats in 1996 at the University of Texas Department of Anatomy and Neurosciences in Galveston, suggested that the drug was clinically safe in moderate doses and that it could be used effectively in pain management for neuropathic patients.

There is evidence that oral administration of Ket will produce fewer side effects than injections. In a few cases these effects can be severe, for example increased salivation and nightmares. Moreover, some practitioners think the oral approach provides as much or more analgesic value than injections. However, Dr. W. S. Kingery at the Physical Medicine and Rehabilitation Service, Veterans Affairs, in Palo Alto, California, found in a late 1997 review of controlled drug tests that there was consistent support for the greater analgesic effectiveness of intravenously administered Ket for PN pain.

Ket can also be used in topical form. A doctor told me that a "compounding" pharmacist can make a preparation of 30–100 mg/ml cream useful for surface application.

Opioids

1. General

Opioids (a.k.a. narcotics) interact with receptors located in the spinal cord and brain, producing **euphoria**, **sedation** and **analgesia**. They alter the mind's perception of painful stimuli by deadening painful impulses transmitted from the peripheral nerves. A significant feature of the analgesia is that it occurs without loss of consciousness.

Many medical professionals are reluctant to prescribe

opioids for PN pain, thinking (or at least claiming) them to be largely ineffective for that purpose. Still, for numerous PN sufferers, they seem to provide the only relief available when pain becomes really overpowering. (This is sometimes referred to as "**break-through pain**" because it seems to break through or overwhelm relief provided by regular medication.)

Opioids are chemically related to **morphine**. Commonly prescribed formulations include morphine itself, **codeine, Dilaudid (hydromorphone), Demerol (meperidine), Dolophine (methadone), Sublimaze (fentanyl), OxyContin (oxycodone)** and **MS Contin (morphine sulfate).**

Often there is a choice as to how opioids will be given. **Orally,** by pill or liquid, is usually preferred because of cost and convenience. **Injections** when called for may be either into a vein, muscle, over the spinal cord or under the skin. Injections produce a quicker result and reduce the amount of opioids required to achieve an analgesic effect. **Implanted pumps** are also used occasionally. Sublimaze is frequently administered by **skin patch** (Duragesic) for around-the-clock medication.

Occasionally the drugs listed above as well as several other opioids are used in **combination** with non-opioid analgesics for PN pain. Included are acetaminophen/oxycodone (trade name **Percocet**), acetaminophen/propoxyphene napsylate **(Darvocet)**, acetaminophen/hydrocodone bitartrate **(Vicodin)**, acetaminophen/codeine **(Tylenol 2, 3, 4),** aspirin/oxycodone hydrochloride and oxycodone terephthalate **(Percodan).**

Often a patient is started on one of these combinations and then if the maximum acceptable ingestion of the non-opioid component is reached before adequate pain relief is obtained he or she is switched to the straight opioid component.

Respiratory depression, which is a decrease in the number of breaths or the depth of breathing, can occur from morphine and other opioid analgesics. Other possible side effects are constipation, nausea and confusion, any of which can significantly interfere with a person's daily life.

[comments re above opioids are not to be considered medical opinions and should not be relied upon as such—always consult your doctor:

(1) After they had injected **morphine** into my spine my pain was cut in half in 2 hours. When the 2nd drug was injected I had no pain within 3 min.—tested by walking around up on the toes and the balls of my feet which hurts me more than anything else. The test was that the 2nd drug would be gone by midnight and from that point on the only help I would have would be from the morphine. I went to noon the 2nd day with very little pain. Jim

(2) Have had a Dr. at the Pain Center and my Internist suggest that after Neurontin, the only answer was **morphine**. Seems too extreme for me with so many options still unexplored. Could some of this reluctance on the part of my Drs. have to do with the particular HMO I'm a member of? Anne

(3) Our society has become so paranoid about illegal drugs that they have forgotten that there are legitimate uses for narcotics. After my pain went beyond the help of all the non-narcotics, plus Tylenol #3 and Darvon, it took me over 2 years to get a doctor to prescribe **morphine**. It was 2

years of pure hell. But my pain specialist explained to me that doctors have a legitimate concern about losing their licenses for prescribing narcotics. Several already have—and their patients were left without any pain control! (And one of them committed suicide!) There have been 2 or 3 exposes on TV about the problem in the past year, and so I hope that the publicity helps. I worry about my doctor being investigated by the DEA—they check pharmacy records to find out which doctors are prescribing the most. The bottom line is that narcotics should be available to chronic pain patients when all other treatments have failed. My doctor told me, when I worried about being on them, that I will probably need them the rest of my life just as diabetics need insulin, or others need blood pressure medicine. All I know is that I went from being almost a vegetable with pain—unable to do anything but watch TV—to being fairly productive again! And I found out I wasn't depressed—I was just IN PAIN. Adele

(4) I have met a pain Dr. who has put me on low doses of **methadone** to control my pain and IT'S WORKING!!!!!!!!! I'm ACTUALLY SLEEPING at night. I take 2 1/2 mg of methadone 4x a day along with my 800mg of Tegretol and my evening dosage of 150 mg Elavil. Adding the methadone to my daily meds has really turned things around for me. I pray that this is not one of those temporary things. Robin

(5) I too have a compassionate doctor. I have lupus and diabetes on top of the PN and AN. The pain was absolutely the worst I have ever experienced and this went on for two years with no help from the pain at all. Depressed, I'll say so—so depressed that living was a chore. Then I happened to see a neurologist who cared. I started out with Vicodin ES but I got so that one every 4–6 hours did nothing which brought on the introduction of the Duragesic Patches [**Sublimaze-fentanyl**]. We started with the 25's went to

50's and are now at 75's but even now I have a lot of break through pain. But I'll take that pain over what I was having to endure before. It sickens me to think of all the people who suffer with chronic pain day in and day out just because of the public's perception of addiction. My heart goes out to any one who does not have a doctor that sees the difference in addiction and real addiction. Nancy K.

(6) For the last three years I have been taking 2 **Percocet** & 1 800 mg Motrin every 4 hours, with Tegretol 400–1200 mg a day, and doxepin at night to help me sleep. This combination makes the pain bearable most of the time. Anon

(7) Well I'm now being awakened at night by pain in my arms and hands. If I move in my sleep in a way that my arms are flexed in any way the pain wakes me up. Then I have to put my arms down at my sides and wait out the pain. The itching and burning in my feet is coming back again also. I find myself having to take at least one more 400mg Neurontin per day just to make life bearable—up to 2000–2400 per day and increasing. I can't believe how fast this is progressing and I'm scared that I'll be unable to maintain much longer. I go for my EMG and NCS on Monday and am going to ask for pain meds—have killer headaches lately—and **Darvocet** just hurts my stomach. Downers which help others sleep cause a speed-like buzz in me so I wonder if Elavil will help or just keep me awake. I read all these posts and garner very little hope . . . sorry this is so long. Diana

(8) I've been to a chronic pain specialist (anesthesiologist) who put me on antidepressants, anticonvulsants and narcotics. My wise GP took me off the narcotics and sent me to a neurologist who continued the antidepressants and the anticonvulsants. I now just take the **Darvocet** (narcotic) to help me when I want to do something special and enjoy myself and to help me make it through the weekends when I'm on my feet more. Velda

(9) I've been living with PN for the last 5 years and have tried everthing under the sun, A-Z. Although taking per-scribed narcotic pain meds might be frowned upon by some, for me it has offered me a way to live pain free and be a functioning member of society. Currently I take OXY-CONTIN 10 mg. 2–3 times per day and **Hydrocodone** 5/500 for breakthrough pain and ELAVIL 100mg. 1 @ bed-time. It is a good idea to experiment with the ELAVIL level, as the dose may not be strong enough at first and it does take time for it to work. And last but not least I give into and acknowledge the pain. It helps if you do not fight it. RELAX. BE CALM. Good luck and God bless. Reba

(10) I, too, am a member of the club from which we'd all love to resign. I take Neurontin 2400mg, Darvocet 3–4 daily, Deseryl, and on really rough days **Vicodin**. My symptoms pretty much mirror those of everyone else. Dov

(11) The pain has been increasing in severity over the past few years, even though my neurologist told my husband and I that it wouldn't get any worse. I am afraid I will end up losing my legs. I currently take 4 **Tylenol** #3 a day as nothing else helps. Julie]

Most of the opioids and opioid combinations listed above have **analgesic effects** lasting only three to four hours except methadone, where the duration is said to ex-tend six to eight hours. **Fentanyl,** currently the only opi-oid commercially available in a **transdermal** form, lasts 72 hours when released through Duragesic skin patches. Another form of fentanyl is a lozenge rubbed inside the cheek where it is quickly absorbed. Called **Actiq**, the opi-oid recently was approved by the FDA for break-through cancer pain. Reportedly, its analgesic effects are 10 times more potent than orally ingested morphine.

OxyContin, one of the newer opioids, is frequently prescribed when an opioid is used for neuropathic pain. It is long acting and needs to be taken only every 8 to 12 hours. **MS Contin**, a drug containing morphine which similarly lasts 8 to 12 hours and is more potent than OxyContin, is also often being used for PN.

[comments re OxyContin and MS Contin are not to be considered medical opinions and should not be relied upon as such—always consult your doctor:

(1) For two years I could not sleep through the night. Neither Neurontin which I still take (2400mg) nor any combinations of about 20 other drugs over a period of 4 years let me sleep. I am now taking **OxyContin** 10mg three times a day and I am sleeping through the night. OxyContin is a narcotic I think, I can't find out much about it. It is in a time release tablet and I have absolutely no side effects. No rushes no highs and after 3 months I have no cravings for it before its time to take it. It just lets me sleep. It has not helped me to wear shoes or walk. I still have the burning feet. I know you may be scared to take this, just use your own judgment and ask a pain doctor about it. Good luck. Jim W.

(2) I went on **OxyContin** about six weeks ago and it has been a real blessing as far as sleep is concerned. For about the past year one to two hours sleep a number of times a day was all I could hope for. With oxycontin I am getting four to six at night, and most important to me, I don't get the drugged feeling I got from regular Percocet. Jim P.

(3) I get relief from taking **OxyContin** which is slow release and it makes a world of difference along with the Neurontin. The oxycontin being 12hr time release I think made a world of difference but my pain management doc

said I would have to take it the rest of my life. Seems the nerves do not die they just keep constantly irritated and it makes me irritable too without the meds!! Angela

(4) The **MS Contin** that I take is a form of morphine. I have no trouble functioning with it but it is not doing much for the pain. It just takes the edge off sometimes. It is also an appetite suppresser and I have lost 62 pounds while on it. Everyone wants to try it!!! But that is not why I am on it. I just wish there was something to take to relieve the pain and burning for awhile. Just 1 hour would sure be nice. That's not asking for much is it??? Lee

(5) My husband has tried the **MS contin** before but the side effects were so bad, dreams, irritability, renal retention, constipation, plus all the rest. His feet have shooting pains, numbness, and are ice cold. Sometimes I wonder how much more he can take. Anon

(6) I was taking **MS Contin** for about 2 mos. before I had back surgery. My doc prescribed it because it is a slow release morphine and does not have Tylenol in it, which most of the other pain killers have and if you take it over a long period of time can cause kidney problems. Actually I did not notice that much of a difference from the class 3 pharmaceuticals. I'm hearing a lot of good things about the morphine pump, which is put in the spinal area. Getting approval seems to be a struggle, but for those who have chronic pain it seems to have improved the quality of life. Jeanne

(7) I take **MS Contin** 30mg. 4 daily, plus xanax and flexeril, and if they just took my MS Contin away I would be in so much pain I don't know what I would do. When I just miss a dose, it makes such a difference in how I feel for the next 8-12 hours. Anon]

The onset of **tolerance**—the need for increased dosages to achieve original effects—often occurs in those taking any of these opioids. The first indication it's developing is when the analgesic effect becomes shorter in duration. Although it was once thought that tolerance limited the effective use of opioids on a long-term basis for pain management, it's now been demonstrated that for most of these drugs there is no arbitrary upper limit of usage.

2. *Image Problems*

Unfortunately, the whole subject of opioids is overlaid with controversy and misunderstandings concerning **drug benefits** versus **dependence**, **tolerance** and **addiction** which could well color a particular professional caretaker's view. As an example, according to a 1992 University of Wisconsin Pain & Policy Study Group report, almost half of 300 doctors surveyed underestimated the relief that pain treatment such as morphine provides to cancer patients.

Many people knowledgeable in this area believe the principal problem here is **not addiction** but rather doctors **under-prescribing** opioids for pain relief, either because they overestimate the addiction risk or because they fear being censured for over prescribing by medical boards or by governmental authorities who oversee the writing of opioid prescriptions.

On the matter of drug addiction, the following is from a story which appeared in a recent issue of *Forbes*:

> "Is a pain-racked patient likely to become an addict? No, said Dr. Dwight Moulin of the University of Western

Ontario in an article in the *Lancet* last year. Morphine, he says, does not produce euphoria in patients with pain, so no craving for anything beyond pain relief ever develops. [Dr. Kathryn] Foley says that in her 30 years as a doctor she has seen only a few cases of morphine addiction among patients with chronic pain. Moulin's study confirmed what others have been saying for a while. A study 20 years ago by Drs. Jose Medina and Seymour Diamond of the Diamond Headache Clinic in Chicago found that only 2 of 2,369 patients exhibited signs of psychological dependence as a result of receiving morphine and other drugs. These studies define addiction fairly narrowly: Only patients who remain dependent on a drug—meaning they crave it after being taken off it—are classified as addicted. But that's not how many doctors in this country see addiction. Doctors believe that a patient who exhibits tolerance and any withdrawal symptoms is addicted. Some patients taking morphine do in fact develop tolerance (meaning they need a higher dose to achieve the same effect) and withdrawal symptoms (like nausea, vomiting and the shakes). But is either of these a reason to make desperately ill people suffer? You can develop tolerance to cortisone, withdrawal problems from caffeine. Morphine's withdrawal symptoms vanish in 12 hours. They are minor compared with those from heroin and alcohol."

The National Institute of Drug Abuse (National Institutes of Health) reported another study examining the potential for drug addiction where long-term therapy was involved. Of 38 chronic pain patients, most of whom had been given opioids for four to seven years, only two reportedly became addicted and they both had a history of drug abuse.

In a public policy statement of April 1997, the American Society of Addiction Medicine (ASAM) offered recommendations and definitions to guide the use of opioid therapy. Here are the key definitions:

"**Physical dependence** on an opioid is a physiologic state in which abrupt cessation of the opioid, or administration of an opioid antagonist, results in a withdrawal syndrome. Physical dependency on opioids is an expected occurrence in all individuals in the presence of continuous use of opioids for therapeutic or for non-therapeutic purposes. It does not, in and of itself, imply addiction.

Tolerance is a form of neuroadaptation to the effects of chronically administered opioids (or other medications) which is indicated by the need for increasing or more frequent doses of the medication to achieve the initial effects of the drug. Tolerance may occur both to the analgesic effects of opioids and to some of the unwanted side effects, such as respiratory depression, sedation, or nausea. The occurrence of tolerance is variable in occurrence, but it does not, in and of itself, imply addiction.

Addiction in the context of pain treatment with opioids is characterized by a persistent pattern of dysfunctional opioid use that may involve any or all of the following:

- adverse consequences associated with the use of opioids
- loss of control over the use of opioids
- preoccupation with obtaining opioids, despite the presence of adequate analgesia. . . .

Individuals who have severe, unrelieved pain may become intensely focused on finding relief for their pain.

Sometimes such patients may appear to observers to be preoccupied with obtaining opioids, but the preoccupation is with finding relief of pain, rather than using opioids per se. This phenomenon has been termed 'pseudoaddiction' in the pain literature ... "

Undoubtedly, in spite of educational efforts there will continue to be misgivings concerning the use of opioids for PN pain, both from patients who fear social disapproval as well as from doctors who either sincerely doubt their benefits or who fear being censured (or even losing their licenses) for over-aggressive prescribing.

3. New Approaches

Because of concerns about addiction as well as about the side effects from opioids, there have been concerted efforts to develop **alternative analgesics**. Some of the work has been supported by the National Institute on Neurological Diseases and Stroke.

One effort has been directed toward the development of **synthetic derivatives** of opioids. It has been known for many years that not only are there receptors throughout the body that respond to opioid substances, but the body itself produces natural opioids which are released during strenuous exercise and in response to stress or pain. Certain compounds derived from these have produced analgesia in rats. It is thought that these compounds might also act to produce analgesia for humans without the opioid side effects. Dr. Lindsay Hough, a principal investigator of synthetic opioid derivatives from the Albany Medical College in New York, told me that patents have already been issued on several of these compounds and that he and his team will be studying these in human neuropathic models in the future.

Recently researchers have discovered that chemicals found in the marijuana plant known as **cannabinoids** relieve certain types of pain. (In fact the name cannabinoids means "like cannabis," the active ingredient in marijuana.) Working with synthetic creations of this chemical, scientists have been able to block pain impulses before they reach the spinal cord. The September 30, 1998, issue of the journal *Nature* detailed experiments conducted on rats. Scientists at the University of California at San Francisco focused on a region deep in the brain which acts as a kind of relay station for pain signals. They found that the synthetic cannabinoid agent they administered acted like morphine in switching on or off certain cells in the same region.

Work is also proceeding to develop "**promoter compounds**" which enhance the pain-relieving effects of opioids in order that smaller doses can be prescribed. The principal aim is to identify non-analgesic drugs which can selectively magnify the beneficial effects of morphine and other opiates. In one study it was demonstrated that **verapamil**, a **calcium channel blocker** used for heart problems, boosted the analgesic effect of morphine and moderated the "high" that is a common side effect of that opioid.

*   *   *

The 1997 review of controlled drug tests by Dr. W. S. Kingery at the Physical Medicine and Rehabilitation Service of Veterans Affairs in Palo Alto, California, previously mentioned in connection with Ket, is an interesting synthesis of studies concerning a number of the non-opioid medications covered in this chapter.

Dr. Kingery analyzed the data found in 72 articles which included 92 controlled drug trials for PN pain using 48 different treatments. According to his analysis there was "consistent support" (in two or more trials) for the analgesic effectiveness of tricyclic antidepressants (Elavil et al.), intravenous and topical lidocaine, intravenous ketamine (Ket), carbamazepine (Tegretol) and topical aspirin. There was only limited support (based on one trial each) for the analgesic effectiveness of oral, topical and epidural clonidine (Catapres) and for subcutaneous ketamine. According to his findings, the trial data were contradictory for mexiletine (Mexitil), phenytoin (Dilantin), topical capsaicin, oral non-steroidal anti-inflammatory medications (Advil et al.) and intravenous morphine. His analysis of the trial *methods*, though, indicated that mexiletine and intravenous morphine were probably effective analgesics for PN pain, while non-steroidals were probably not. He reported that studies indicated codeine, magnesium chloride, propranolol, lorazepam, and intravenous phentolamine all failed to provide analgesia in single trials. Dr. Kingery found there were no long-term data supporting the analgesic effectiveness of *any* drug and the etiology of the neuropathy did not predict treatment outcome.

Having come across this study, I would have felt derelict in not bringing it to your attention. Nevertheless, based on anecdotal evidence as well as other studies

in this chapter, one might well question some of its findings and conclusions. In any event, I hope it would not
discourage any PNers (or their doctors) from trying particular medications which Kingery believes are not well
substantiated in the literature. As has been said before,
different things work for different people. The various
comments in this chapter should offer ample proof of
that.

Chapter 4

Other Medical Therapies

There are a number of ways PN pain has been treated in addition to the administration of medications. Some of these are quite orthodox and have solid science behind them. Others where the science is thought to be more questionable (or outright mysterious) are dealt with in the next chapter concerning "alternative therapies."

Not all the treatments discussed in this chapter, however, have to do solely with the alleviation of pain. Plasmapheresis, immunosuppressants and IVIg, discussed below, seek to overcome other problems affecting certain PNers as well as pain.

Hematological Treatments

The therapies dealt with under this heading are directed mainly to the **autoimmune** condition known as CIDP (**chronic inflammatory demyelinating poly-**

neuropathy). In this situation the body's own immune system mistakenly attacks the myelin sheath protecting nerves. Consequences of CIDP include paralysis or weakness of arms or legs, respiratory problems and burning sensations. GBS (**Guillain Barre syndrome**) is another autoimmune PN condition with even more severe consequences, including the possibility of total paralysis or respiratory failure. The hematological treatments covered here, which deal with these autoimmune conditions, seem to be well accepted among practitioners.

1. Plasmapheresis

This is a procedure, as noted, targeted principally at immune-mediated PN and used generally in more severe cases. Under this procedure the plasma of the blood—the fluid part—is removed from blood cells by a **cell separator**. This is done either by spinning the blood at a high speed to separate the fluid from the cells or by filtering the blood through a membrane with holes so small that only the plasma can make it through. The removed fluid or plasma contains the antibodies believed to attack the myelin sheath in cases of CIDP. The red and white blood cells are then returned to the body along with other fluids.

Usually the treatment takes several hours and is uncomfortable but generally not painful. The number of treatments varies but an average is six to ten over a two to ten week period. A small tube or catheter is placed in a large arm vein and another in the opposite hand or foot. Blood is transmitted to the separator from the first

tube and the separated blood cells together with the replacement fluids are returned in the other.

The most common side effect is said to be a drop in
blood pressure, experienced as faintness or dizziness, and
occasionally sweating or abdominal cramps. Overall, however, plasmapheresis is considered to be well tolerated.

*[comments re plasmapheresis are not to be consid-
ered medical opinions and should not be relied upon
as such- always consult your doctor:*

(1) I have had 17 **plasmapheresis** treatments, and I am
definitely seeing some improvement. I have three more to
go. It IS expensive, but my insurance is paying for it. The
key is having a doctor who knows how to deal with insurance companies! I am now on Methotrexate, but it's making me sick, so I don't know if I'll be staying on it. Doctors
said plasmapheresis must be followed by some type of
chemo. Jenny

(2) I am now on **plasmapheresis** treatments. I am getting
eight treatments and then going to be assessed to see what
is next. So far I had 4 plasmapheresis treatments and I notice a big difference. Now I don't get as weak and have a lot
more stamina. Even the pain is better. I don't know if it
will last, only time will tell. Anon

(3) Yes, I'm getting **plasmapheresis**. I had four treatments each month (March—May) on a Mon Wed Fri Mon.
The first time, it took almost three weeks before I got relief,
but it's been non stop since then. I haven't received any
this month; we're trying to see how long I can go between
sessions. It's heaven to be "back to my life." I haven't taken
pain pills since March. The disease is still there, but the
pain is liveable. It's great to be off drugs. It's starting to go
the other way now—slowly. So I guess it's time to call the

neurologist back again. The only side effect that I've had is about every fourth time, my blood pressure "bottoms" out and they have to make me lay down flat. It takes about two hours for my blood pressure to go back into normal range. Normally, it only takes an hour for the treatment. It helps to have good veins, but they can put in a port. Drink as much water as possible, as it makes your veins stand up and makes the process go smoother. Before this I had IVIg, which gave me six weeks of pain relief, but the next treatments didn't work. I have a friend, who has CIDP and had plasmapheresis for two years before it stopped working. He's getting IVIg now & having good results. My PN is idiopathic sensory PN of the small fibers. Good Luck. Cathy]

2. Immunosuppressant Medications

The improvement which a patient achieves through plasmapheresis (which can be significant) generally lasts no longer than four to eight weeks. This is thought to be because the antibodies will eventually return unless the patient is placed on other **immunosuppressive** therapy such as **Imuran (azathioprine)** or **prednisone**. This suppression of the immune system also gives the body a chance to re-myelinate the damaged and frayed nerves.

Imuran's principal "on label" use is for the treatment of patients who have kidney transplants. However, it has been found quite effective as an immunosuppressant in the treatment of CIDP, both in conjunction with plasmapheresis and as used alone. Side effects of Imuran usage include the possible serious lowering of the white blood cell count, resulting in an increased risk of infection. Imuran can also cause liver toxicity, nausea, vomiting and loss of appetite.

Imuran is often initiated at 50 mg per day with the dosage gradually increased to 150 mg daily, depending on side effects and pain relief obtained.

Prednisone, a **synthetic corticosteroid** (in its natural form a substance produced by the adrenal glands located adjacent to the kidneys) with potent anti-inflammatory properties, is often used in combination with Imuran. It also acts as an immunosuppressant.

The initial dosage of prednisone reportedly varies from 5 mg to 60 mg per day depending on the patient and the severity of the condition. The available clinical information emphasizes dosage needs to be individualized based upon the response of the particular patient. After a favorable response is noted, through adjustments where necessary, this information states the proper maintenance dosage should then be determined by decreasing the initial dosage in small amounts until the lowest dosage which will maintain an adequate response is reached. If after long-term therapy the drug is to be discontinued, it is recommended that it be withdrawn gradually rather than abruptly. In fact an abrupt withdrawal can cause serious problems, even death.

Possible side effects of prednisone use, which may be severe in some situations, include a long list: diabetes induction, hypertension, gastritis/ulcers, osteoporosis, insomnia, depression, tremors, muscle weakness, fluid retention, glaucoma, cataracts, weight gain and fat redistribution.

A neurologist told me that small doses of Imuran and prednisone when taken together can produce the same result as a larger dose of either taken alone, requiring less medication in the aggregate. Another benefit of this approach, he said, is that the unwelcome side effects of the two are sufficiently different that the overall potentially harmful consequences of immunosuppressant medication for the patient can be significantly lessened.

Another synthetic corticosteroid, **Decadron (dexamethasone)**, is sometimes but less often prescribed.

[comments re Imuran and prednisone are not to be considered medical opinions and should not be relied upon as such- always consult your doctor:

(1) I tried **Imuran** for a few months, gradually working up to 150mg. a day. I saw no change in my PN, and after a couple of months it started to affect my liver. Tell your friend to make sure her doctor does liver function tests (blood) at least once a month, as Imuran is absorbed through the liver, and can cause damage. Anon

(2) I have been on 200 mgs daily of **Imuran** since my last relapse in February/97. So far, so good. I am also taking **prednisone** (I am down to 12 1/2 alternating with 5). I have had CIDP for 16 years, so for most of those years "it" had no name nor protocol. In the last four years I have tried gamma globulin (worked great for a year and then stopped). Then at each relapse I would have plasmapheresis, which brings me back to life. I had tried Imuran once before and my system could not handle it. Now, thankfully, my system is cooperating. Yes there are side-effects, as with everything else we could take for CIDP. Every month my neuro does blood tests to check for liver damage, etc. For me it is had been a life saver, I can walk! Lynda

(3) I'm starting to get those "burning" sensations all over, in fleeting jabs, and I don't like it!! This disease is progressing faster than a lightening bolt, and I can't do anything to stop it! I'm taking **prednisone** and **Imuran**, but

obviously, they aren't doing anything to "stave off" the disease, as my doctor hoped they would. Jenny

(4) I have had neuropathy for 3 yrs. I am also a 4th generationer to have asthma When I have an attack I am put on **prednisone**. The stuff works wonders for my feet, but it causes me to become diabetic. Without realizing it my blood sugar rose to 800. NOT GOOD!!!!!!!!!!! Prednisone also can cause some type of blindness, I'm not sure how but my allergist requires me to have my eyes checked, if I've had to be on prednisone for a couple of months. Anon

(5) My doctor diagnosed my PN saying that my antibodies were eating away at the nerve sheaths. He started me out at 20 mg **prednisone** for one month and then 40 mg the next month which is almost over. Within two weeks I noticed that the pain had dropped at least 50% and even though I don't get to sleep until around 0500–0700 the pain is something I can live with. My fingers seem to continue to get worse (like raw without skin) but my feet have improved tremendously. Martin

(6) Do not skip **prednisone** dosage. The prednisone stops the body temporarily from producing adrenal hormones and if you stop the prednisone that is replacing it, you could have heart problems and failure. Please keep your dosage on time til the doctor tapers you off. Very important. Tim

(7) I have CIDP also. I have gone through many treatments. Like your mother, plasma brings me back to life. I have been on **Imuran** and **prednisone** for a year without a relapse. I am now on 5 mg of prednisone daily. I know prednisone is not something I would like to take all my life BUT after suffering with this "weird" disability for 17 years, I am happy to be able to function. I was also taking gamma globulin for a year but unfortunately it "wore off." Best wishes. Lynda

(8) Hi all. I just wanted to relay this bit of happening. My friend, Vickie, that has PN, well, her doctor put her on 20 mg. of **prednisone**. She was on it for 11 days when she had a rare, but severe reaction to it. We thought she was having a stroke. She couldn't walk, talk or swallow. Her left side was numb. The doctors at two different ER's both said it was the prednisone. So, she is off of it now. And, back to normal except her memory is bad as a result, but that will repair itself within a couple of weeks. It's too bad, too, because it was helping her with her leg pain and spasms at night. Anon]

A chemotherapy medication called **Cytoxan** (generic is **cyclophosphamide**) is also sometimes used with plasmapheresis (as well as with IVIg, covered next). This is another immunosuppressive in its own right and reportedly inhibits the growth of rapidly reproducing cells by interfering with the processing of their **DNA**. Cytoxan is a powerful drug with side effects which can be significant such as urinary bleeding, sterility, anemia and cardiac problems. Further, usage of this drug can itself pose a long-term risk of certain types of cancer. Medical practitioners advise that a person taking this drug, similarly to prednisone, needs to be **closely monitored** by his or her caretaker. Plenty of fluids are also advised.

Still other immunosuppressants include cyclosphorin and tacrolimus. The attending physician often may be required to try several before finding the immunosuppressant that works best and can be tolerated.

[comments re Cytoxan are not to be considered medical opinions and should not be relied upon as such-always consult your doctor:

(1) I was diagnosed with CIDP and was treated with prednisone, gamma globulin injections and chemotherapy (**Cytoxan**). Of the three the IVIg was the most effective with very few side affects. Prednisone made me much weaker and the Cytoxan made my hair fall out and left me vulnerable to sore throats (I get strep throat easily) so I stopped taking it. Mary

(2) My doctor's recommendation was to do an additional plasma exchange, and at the completion of this exchange include chemotherapy which would involve an infusion of **Cytoxan**. The intent was to eliminate the production of white blood cells which would retard or stop the IGM protein production and therefore eliminate the problem. Started the 2nd Plasma exchange on the 12th of Sept. Completed exchange on the 18th, received Cytoxan on the 19th. The 20th felt pretty good—well enough to play a little football with my teenage son (very little). Sunday the 21st, the quality of life changed drastically. Went to get out of bed and fell. Numbness at this point had traveled up to my ankles. Ankles to mid calf felt good. From mid calf to just above my knees, felt weak and numb. Both hands up to my elbows were also numb and tingling. My hands to my touch felt like putting your hands on a peg board. They felt dry and callused. Strange feeling. Very hard to describe. Ended up being hospitalized on the 28th. Russell

(3) I have tried Chemo (**Cytoxan**) and had to stop because of side effects (bladder). It was apparently doing no good since I tried it for 6 weeks with no obvious improvement. It involved taking a blood test each week. Anon

(4) Two and a half years ago one of my doctors prescribed **cytoxan** for my neuropathy. . . . Over a three month period I received 15 doses of cytoxan, first 720mg., then 680 mg. I became weaker during this therapy, and blood tests indicated it was not having the desired effect, so it was discon-

tinued. The therapy that has been most beneficial for me has been infusions of IVIg (gamma globulin); I'm currently receiving 30 g. a week. James]

3. IVIg

IVIg is a high dose solution of proteins called **gamma globulins** which contain **antibodies** providing immunity against disease. The gamma globulins are manufactured from pooled, donated blood. In IVIg administered for CIDP and GBS, the gamma globulin antibodies are thought to block the action of the antibodies causing the myelin damage.

IVIg is administered **intravenously**. Each infusion takes three to six hours. At the beginning of therapy an induction dose is usually given over two to five days. Subsequently, maintenance doses are ordinarily given monthly for a limited period of time.

The IVIg procedure can be performed in conjunction with the use of **steroids**, **methotrexate** and other immunosuppressants such as prednisone, as well as following plasmapheresis. It can also be used with antibiotics if the patient is suffering from an infection. The procedure may be accomplished in a hospital or clinic, at a doctor's office or with proper supervision, by the patient at home.

A few patients who take IVIg treatments have experienced severe side effects. These have included hepatitis, renal failure and excessive clotting. Consequently, it has been suggested that patients be screened by special blood tests before undertaking these treatments.

Positive results for IVIg have been reported in studies

which were both double-blind (neither the CIDP patients nor the administrator knowing who were receiving the globulins and who were receiving the placebos) and cross over (the patients receiving the IVIg and placebo were reversed mid-way through the studies). Anecdotal reports as well as double blind studies for the use of IVIg in CIDP and GBS cases also are mostly favorable.

In a 1997 study performed at the Service de Neurologie et Maladies Neuromusculaires, in Marseilles, France, 18 patients (15 men, 3 women; age range 30 to 71 years, mean 45.8 years) with multifocal motor neuropathy (i.e., a particular type of neuropathy affecting more than one nerve), were treated with high dosage IVIg—400 mg daily for three to five days. Clinical improvement was noted in 12 of the 18. Often, though, these patients needed repeated courses of IVIg to maintain the improvement. The infusions were terminated for two without signs of relapse after a year. The results indicated to the researchers that there were long-term benefits using IVIg in multifocal motor neuropathy but also that the benefits were sometimes just transient.

The major concerns about this therapy at the present are availability and expense. When this was written there was reportedly a world-wide shortage of gamma globulin. Cost estimates for a single infusion range from $8,000 to $26,000 though it is often covered by insurance or Medicaid.

[comments re IVIg are not to be considered medical opinions and should not be relied upon as such— always consult your doctor:

(1) I, too, have CIDP and am taking **IVIg** plus prednisone. The IVs didn't work for me until they were moved closer together. At under 4 weeks between the last two treatments I showed remarkable recovery. It's been 6 weeks since my last IV and tomorrow I start another two treatments. The Dr. hopes it will put me "over the top" for awhile, at least. Personal needs seem to vary. Ting

(2) After 6 mos. of prednisone with no improvement, my Dr. is weaning me off. However, when I thought I was doomed to keep failing, I started **IVIg** and after the correct interval between treatments was found, I began to improve markedly. If things continue and I regain some muscle I will begin to feel human again. Alice

(3) I had gamma globulin [**IVIg**] treatments last week, five days consecutively. Each day I received 30 grams. It comes ten grams to a bottle, so of course that means three bottles. I understand it is expensive but the problem I had was that there is a shortage of gamma globulin in Boston and the head of the blood bank has to "sign off" on each bottle and decide who needs it the most. Fortunately it was approved and I did have five treatments. So far I haven't noticed any change, but the doctor in the blood bank said I shouldn't expect to see anything for approximately two weeks. I had the first two infusions as an in-patient. I was told that a very small percentage of people are allergic to the gamma globulin but that if you are allergic you can die from it so they wanted me in the hospital where I could be helped if there was a reaction. Fortunately there wasn't. I was also told (I ask lots of questions) that the gamma globulin is helpful for less than 50 percent of the people receiving it. Not too encouraging. The plan now is for me to receive one infusion a month for six months. Doris

(4) Yes, I would recommend a nerve biopsy in trying to identify the cause. I had one and it showed swelling, white blood cell infiltration and small nerve fiber loss. This led

to a diagnosis of small fiber neuropathy being probably caused by an over-reactive immune system (like an auto-immune disease) where the nerves are being acted on by my own body. My first type of treatment was high dose prednisone which has not worked well. Now, I am beginning a trial of **IV gamma-globulin** infusions because my neurologist feels the neuropathy is progressing faster than the prednisone treatment could react. There is not much clinical evidence to show the IVIg treatment will work, but its a "shot" at trying. I'll try anything to halt or end the onslaught of my disease and the daily experience of pain/disability. Brian

(5) I, too, have undergone **IVIg**. After six months of prednisone with no appreciable results IVIg was recommended. It was scheduled close to home. (We live in the country and travel 250 miles RT to the neurologist) so it was not time consuming (30 miles away. A piece of cake.) Five days in a row about four hours each day. (The first day was about four and a half hours because they wanted to start slowly.) No problems whatsoever and no apparent side effects although I was briefed on the potential. They left the needle (shunt) in the arm all week and just covered it with an Ace bandage. It was actually an interesting experience. There were chairs for about thirty five patients and they were all occupied most of the time. We actually got interesting dialogue going. I cannot say if there was any benefit to the treatment but emotionally I want to say it helped. I may do it again and if cost is not a factor can recommend it without hesitation. Five days—four hours each—about $12000.00 all covered by my insurance. Hey, it's an option. You should look at everything except spinal taps and nerve biopsy. No more of that stuff for me. Keep the spirit up and good luck. Stan

(6) Yes I had **immunoglobulin** treatments. I got 5 in a row once a month for 5 months. Yes it helped it helped a lot. The side effects I had left a bad taste in my mouth and a

very upset stomach. I found if I got up and moved and kept doing something for an hour or so I felt fine. It was worth it but after I was finished with the treatments all my problems came back. Now my doctor tells me gamma globulin is hard to get and only the most needy will get it. Yes I would take it again if it were available. Lyle

(7) Received four **IVIg** treatments and I broke out in a rash all over except on my face, very itchy and my hands, arms and chest were the worst. I had to go on prednisone. Went off it last week and now my hands are starting to break out again. I also was on Benadryl and Lidex Cream. Needless to say I can't have any further treatments due to the reaction. Kay

(8) I have been on **IVIg** for 5 months now and it has worked well. I have had 4 treatments of 46 grams a day for 5 consecutive days spaced 4 weeks a part. I have regained complete usage of my hands and my legs/feet get better with each treatment. I'm taking some time in between treatments now to see how long I can go before back sliding. Anon

(9) I was released from the hospital yesterday. My second of 2 [**IVIg**] treatments finished at 1:40 AM Sunday (yesterday morning). I received two 50 gram treatments, 10% solution at 63 CC's an hour. Each treatment was 8 hours. I was pre-medicated with two Tylenol and 1 benadril. Already my left hand is straighter and wrist flexion stronger. I am so amazed! I LOVE my new doctors. Both went to Columbia and were students of Dr. Latov. I asked many questions during my stay and truly believe I was misdiagnosed for years! Well, not to worry anymore! Elizabeth]

4. Comparison of Treatments

Neurologists at St. Elizabeth's Medical Center of Boston made an attempt to determine which of the three principal treatments for CIDP and GBS discussed above—plasmapheresis, immunosuppressants or IVIg—worked best. They conducted a retrospective analysis of 67 cases for this purpose. The investigators concluded, as described in a 1997 MedReport from the Center, that all three were similar in their effectiveness. The response rate was between 40 and 60% with any one therapy. However, the investigators discovered that half the patients who did not respond to the first therapy (it didn't make any difference which was used first) improved with a second and that one-third of those who did not respond to the second did so with the third. The over-all result was that about 70% of the patients were benefited by one of the three therapies.

Nerve-Based Treatments

1. Nerve Blocks

Nerve blocks have been used in both diagnostic and treatment procedures for many years. Their use in the treatment of chronic pain, particularly where there has been an injury to a nerve root or a nerve, is now a well established practice although some medical professionals think they should be reserved until the time when pain seems so great as to be otherwise untreatable.

The procedure involves **injection by needle** of either a **local anesthetic** or a **neurolytic** (nerve destructive) agent into a peripheral nerve in order to decrease or eliminate nerve activity. The administration of a local anesthetic such as **lidocaine** or **bupivacaine**, sometimes with a steroid like **cortisone**, is often done first to assess the likely effect of a more permanent block. This **initial block** usually lasts for a few hours, long enough to allow assessment of the functional impact to be expected from the neurolytic block.

(German physicians commonly are said to administer anesthetic injections into various sites such as nerves and acupuncture points [discussed in the next chapter] under a procedure they call "**neural therapy**." These physicians are reported to believe the injections restore electrical conductivity throughout the body and permit healing to occur. See *The Alternative Medicine Handbook,* pp. 190–91, W. W. Norton & Co., 1998. Nevertheless, many practitioners have serious reservations about this procedure.)

Peripheral nerve destruction is intended to provide a long lasting block to pain signals. This is accomplished through the injection of **ethanol**, **phenol** or another neurolytic agent into the nerve at sites where a local anesthetic was used first to provide a functional assessment.

The injected neurolytic agent destroys many of the nerve fibers with which it comes in contact, in effect "thinning" out the nerve. The relief from pain following this procedure often is said to last months, in some cases years, but rarely permanently. The reason given for the limited effect is that, unlike brain or spinal cord cells, peripheral nerves are often able to **regenerate** (but obviously not completely or perfectly or we wouldn't have our pain problems). A special caution should be noted here:

there is said to be some possibility that a nerve already troubled by PN could be further damaged by the phenol or other chemicals used in the block instead of being totally suppressed, perhaps causing more pain than before. Some practitioners believe this could be resolved (hopefully) by a repetition of the procedure.

In two more radical techniques a neurosurgeon will sometimes cut a nerve close to the spinal cord (**rhizotomy**) or bundles of nerves in the spinal cord itself (**cordotomy**) in order to permanently block nerve pathwaves which relay pain impulses to the brain. Obviously these procedures involve major surgery.

Side effects from nerve blocks are generally not considered significant. Headaches, hypotension and respiratory depression are said to occur sometimes but only rarely.

Most of the experience with regard to nerve blocks comes from physicians working with cancer patients. It has been reported that anywhere from 50 to 80% of cancer victims who receive such blocks may benefit from them. However, if the following comments can be believed, nerve blocks may be less effective for those with peripheral neuropathy.

[comments re nerve blocks are not to be considered medical opinions and should not be relied upon as such—always consult your doctor:

(1) I had 4 lumbar/thoracic **nerve blocks** at UCLA Pain Management Center. They only helped for a few hours at the most. They're very expensive and who wants to go through that every week. I've heard nothing but bad re-

ports on nerve cuts. So far, finding the right medicine combination seems the best bet. Don't look for cures, just insist on treating the pain. We all pray that the cure is around the corner, but waiting for it everyday can be a crazy maker. Velda

(2) I've been given several **nerve blocks**. My first one lasted 2 weeks and my last one numbed me for 3 days. It seems the more I have them, the bigger the tolerance my body has for them. A word of caution, about the nerve cutting. You need to see an orthopedic surgeon for that (at least that was the type dr. I saw for it). The dr. spoke a lot about phantom pain. He said that not everyone becomes pain free after nerve cutting. Me, personally I would rather have real pain than phantom pain. I think phantom pain would drive me crazy. It is hard enough getting the drs. to believe that PN has real pain. Robin

(3) I had two **nerve blocks**. In one the needles were inserted around my ankles—several "sticks." Two, the single "stick" was made in my back along the spinal cord (not in it). The ankle shot helped that foot for about 4 hours. The shot in the back did nothing at all. Sorry for this news. Jim W.

(4) I had sympathetic **nerve block** procedure done at Downstate Medical Center Pain clinic—without any success. The doctors gave up on me. They couldn't figure out a course of treatment for the burning pain I have on my right foot for the past 3 plus years (after laminectomy). Sorry. James

(5) I too have suffered [from migraine headaches] for 17 years or more. I have been medicated and nothing has helped. I went to a pain doctor who works with University of Chicago who tested me for the possibility of a permanent **nerve block**. The temporary test lasts a month if it works . . . it did for me. I had a permanent double nerve block

done last Christmas. It has given me my life back. I am off all but Imitrex (which I rarely take anymore). The block doesn't get rid of the headaches or symptoms, but it blocks the excruciating [PN] pain. I feel pressure instead, but what a difference. I can usually take a few aspirin and I am ok. When the pressure is bad, I use the shots. I was taking tons of Imitrex before, since the block, I have only used it 3 times and it has been 6 months. My insurance covered the costs. I also did biofeedback training which helped me stay off some of the symptoms if I could raise my body temp when it was dropping. Bob

(6) I have suffered for about 10 years now. The last two years have been really bad as far as pain goes. I take 6 Neurontin a day, also 4 Ultram and Tylenol and Motrin. The things I have found for relief are as follows. Massage, hot tub swimming, using my TENS unit. I'm trying something brand new to me: chelation therapy. The idea is that it will clear out some of my clogged up arteries in my legs and feet giving me better circulation and free me from the frozen feet that I usually suffer from. I will let you know if this is the solution for less pain. I sure hope so. I have tried so many things over the years that have not helped at all most of which insurance does not cover. Magnetic insoles, acupuncture, physical therapy, probably the worst was shots given in my lower back under anesthesia, a **block** into the sympathetic nerves. It was a series of four shots. You have to go into the hospital each time. No relief. The doctor wants to implant something in my back to reduce pain. I don't think so!!!!! Sherman]

2. Direct Nerve Stimulation

The best known means of stimulating nerves directly in order to alleviate PN pain is "**transcutaneous elec-**

trical nerve stimulation" or TENS. This procedure refers to the use of a battery-powered device about the size of a small transistor radio which transmits electrical current through the skin to underlying nerves. Electrodes are placed at specific sites near or at the location of the perceived pain. The device is then turned on and the current intensity increased until a slight tingling sensation is felt. (Both the frequency and voltage of the electrical current are considered important.) According to its proponents, after 40 minutes or so the pain is significantly reduced.

There are several mechanisms of TENS action which are postulated. It supposedly is able to **stimulate fast conducting nerves** which travel to the spinal cord, closing the gate of entry before the pain message from the slower pain conducting nerves gets there. Also it is thought that TENS **suppresses the electrical firing** which occurs at nerve endings producing pain. Further, it's speculated that an **analgesic block** is produced in the central nervous system and that TENS triggers the release of **endorphins**, mentioned before—chemical substances with powerful analgesic properties occurring naturally in the brain.

One manufacturer of these devices (and there are many) claims a success rate of 85% with the use of TENS. Others point out that their units are **non-invasive** and say they eliminate or reduce the need for drugs. They contend the only problems are possible skin irritations where the electrodes are placed.

As to clinical validations, one study on TENS conducted at the University of Washington simply related that it was "better than placebo for PN neuropathy." (Possibly not *quite* as strong a statement on efficacy as the device manufacturers would like to have seen!) Another study which was summarized in a December 1995 issue of *Pain* found the average pain decrease due to peripheral nerve injury was 75% during stimulation sessions. Reportedly, the duration of relief often outlasted the period of stimulation by several hours, occasionally for days or even weeks. Further daily stimulation carried out at home by patients was found to sometimes provide gradually increasing relief over additional periods of weeks or months.

A study reported in the May–June 1998 issue of the *Journal of Foot & Ankle Surgery*, attempted to assess the longer term benefits of TENS. Seventy six patients with diabetic neuropathy were surveyed who had been using a TENS unit for about one and a half years on average. Forty-one or 76% reported an approximate 44% improvement in their neuropathic pains based on subjective criteria.

A study performed at the University of Southern California Medical Center and reported in a November 1997 issue of *Diabetes Care*, evaluated the efficacy of TENS for 31 people with Type 2 diabetes having peripheral neuropathy. The patients were divided into two groups, one receiving TENS and a control group getting a "sham" treatment. All patients treated each of their lower extremities for 30 minutes daily for four weeks at home. (Nine from the control group participated for a second period, during which they received TENS therapy.) Neuropathic symptoms improved in five (38%) patients in the control or placebo group, suggesting a procedure-related placebo effect (i.e., the power of suggestion mentioned before). In the TENS group symptomatic improvement was seen in 15 (83%) cases, and post-treatment pain scores were considerably lower than in the control group, seeming to indicate a substantial treatment effect over and above any placebo influence. Moreover, later TENS treatments decreased pain scores significantly in the nine patients who had first received sham treatments.

Another interesting report, also from researchers at the University of Southern California Medical Center, was published in a September 1998 issue of *Diabetes Care*. Twenty six people with diabetic neuropathy were placed on Elavil. After four weeks, 60 percent reported some pain relief, averaging a 26 percent reduction using standard pain measures. Then, in addition, the participants received either real or sham electrotherapy, similar but reportedly not identical to TENS. Among those receiving both Elavil and electrotherapy, 85 percent reported improvement, and their pain scores dropped 66 percent from baseline.

Generally a TENS unit can either be rented for short periods of time or purchased by a patient who intends to use it long term. Most insurance carriers appear to be willing to pay for the rental or the purchase.

Electromedical Products International, Inc. (located in Mineral Wells, Texas; 1-800-FOR-PAIN), is marketing a device using what they call **"microcurrent therapy"** (METS). The company claims its unit, which employs lower electric currents than typical TENS units as well as self-adhesive probes and electrodes, provides longer lasting relief than do TENS devices.

Another company, Prizm Medical, Inc., manufactures a two ounce electrical stimulator called the **Micro-Z** which delivers a tiny current through garments. The socks, gloves and sleeves which are also marketed by the company, are made of nylon, dacron and silver and can be worn during the day or at night. The key to Micro-Z is said to be that "electrotherapy energy" is delivered to the entire area where the garment meets the skin. Prizm claims the stimulator "provides mild, therapeutic relief of pain, reduces swelling and increases blood circulation." (Prizm can be reached at 1-800-447-4422.)

I also came across several studies on the somewhat related subject of **"spinal cord stimulation"** or SCS. (It's like the military, everyone in medicine seems to use acronyms.) This is a relatively new surgical procedure accomplished through the implanting of electrodes near the spinal cord. In one investigation (at the University of Saskatchewan), among 30 patients diagnosed with peripheral neuropathy, 19 reported relief of pain and had their electrodes permanently implanted. At an average of 87 months follow up, 14 indicated long-term success in pain control.

In another SCS study at Walton Diabetes Centre, Walton Hospital in Liverpool, England, (reported in the medical journal *Lancet*, December 21, 1996) involving 10 diabetic patients with PN who had not responded to conventional treatments, 8 reported significant pain abatement and had their units permanently implanted. Six said they continued to gain pain relief after their implantations and claimed to rely on the stimulator as their sole source of treatment. One interesting aspect of the study was that the patients were doing treadmill exercises during the entire period to assess their exercise tolerance. According to the investigators, all showed an increase in the ability to exercise with the median improvement being 150% over the six months of the study.

The most recent investigation I found was conducted at the Department of Neurological Surgery, University of Pittsburgh, in 1998 (reported in the July 1998 issue of *Neurological Research*). Twenty-seven patients with intractable pain (one with peripheral neuropathy) were selected for the administration of spinal cord stimulation. These had all been pre-screened under what was said to have been a rigorous protocol which eliminated people with psychological and behavioral problems and those where corrective surgery might have been a better alternative. Of the 27 initially in the study, 24 chose to have stimulators implanted after a three-day trial period during which they were connected to an external stimulation source. After an average 21 month follow-up, 22 of the 24 were said to have experienced pain reduction from the internal stimulator. All 22 indicated they would choose to receive an electric stimulator again if given the opportunity.

Another method for controlling pain through the introduction of an electric current involves implanting electrodes directly in the brain. It is sometimes used for advanced forms of cancer. (I did not find any specific reference to its use for neuropathic pain, perhaps not too surprising considering the somewhat radical nature of the procedure.) Once the implant is made the patient determines when and how much stimulation is needed by operating an external transmitter. Patients who have used this reportedly say their "pain melts away" and that they experience no loss of mental functions.

[comments re TENS and SCS are not to be considered medical opinions and should not be relied upon as such—always consult your doctor:

(1) The **TENS** unit is the only thing that relieves my pain. If I don't wear it, it is an effort to walk 300 feet to the mailbox. When I wear it, I can walk more than a mile. This weekend I walked all over the state fairgrounds. I hate wearing it with the electrodes, all the wires and having the thing clipped to my pants, but until something better comes along, I will continue to use it. Marcia

(2) Medicare gave me a free 30 day trial of a **TENS** unit and I didn't find it helpful enough to have them buy it for me. Jim

(3) I tried a **TENS** unit. After a few minutes, I would end up with muscles contracting every time I used them or the thing went "on." I think it distracted me from the pain more than blocking the pain, if that makes any sense at all.

A doctor once told me that if something works, go for it. It doesn't really matter how it works even if it is a placebo affect. That was probably the only good piece of advice that doctor gave me. Maureen

(4) I do have a **TENS** unit given to me by my brother-in-law who is a pharmacist in business for himself. I find that it runs hot and cold. Sometimes it does give me relief, however as soon as I remove the unit, that's the end of the relief. Sometimes it doesn't help at all. It runs about $400 a unit and for that kind of money I think you should get more relief from pain for hours after using it, so who knows. But if you could borrow one and see for yourself before buying that would be best. They are confining as you have to attach nodes to your feet and you can't really move from place to place. I haven't used mine for an age, but I guess I'll try it again, however, my neuropathy is worse than it was when I last used it (last year some time) so I'm not expecting much. Debra

(5) We got a **TENS** unit for my mother today and are trying it now. I have seen some of you on here questioning about placement. A physical therapist hooked up my mother's and explained about placement, he gave us a sheet with diagrams, BUT, he stressed the importance of experimenting with different locations. He said that he had seen people receive wonderful pain relief from TENS units. He told us not to give up after the first day, that many times people will think it is not going to work for them but through experimentation they will find their "magical spot." He also said to experiment with the settings. Shawn

(6) I used one (**TENS** unit) for two years before getting PN. It's sort of like electronic aspirin. There is a new type of unit now that's called microcurrent tens (**METS**) and you don't really feel that shock sensation with this new unit. The trou-

ble is that it doesn't seem to do anything for the symptoms of PN. It does seem to have some effect on arthritis, but you can only use them for up to a couple of hours per day. The new unit costs about $750, and some insurance providers don't like the idea of paying for a "magic box." Anon

7) I have been using the Alpha Stim unit (**METS)** since January 94 and have had great results. I was diagnosed with peripheral neuropathy in both legs in the spring 93, at which time I was put on a variety of pain killers. The pain was so bad I could hardly walk, much less sleep. I eventually ended up on Opium substitutes that had me in a haze most of the time and unable to hold food down. Upon receiving the Alpha Stim unit I was able to slowly wean myself off of the drugs and have been drug free since January 94, in addition to gaining back 30 lbs I had lost due to the effects of the drugs I was on. Paul

(8) I've never used a TENS unit but I did a trial with a **Spinal Cord Stimulator**. The trial worked, helped with the pain, but I can't get the permanent one since I take Coumadin due to minor strokes. The SCS sends a "buzzing" down into your legs and/or feet depending on how you set it up. Shirley

(9) If you're referring to **Spinal Cord Stimulator**, don't do it. Only good for one nerve, highly discouraged by major medical in 41centers in Midwest. Quint [author's note—interesting contrast between reports such as this and the quite positive trial results noted above. This is purely a personal opinion but it seems to me SCS is worth investigating if one has continuing, intense, unbearable pain with a long term opioid regimen perhaps being the only alternative.]

Chapter 5

Alternative Treatments

The term "alternative medicine" means different things to different people. To some it may conjure up thoughts of occult therapies practiced far off in a tent. To others it means just getting back to nature. Most of us think of alternative medicine, though, simply as treatments out of medicine's mainstream—treatments that have a chance of working for us where others haven't.

Sometimes our willingness to try one or more of these is prompted by a (well-founded) suspicion that continued use of any medication, even those sold over-the-counter like most NSAIDs, isn't the best thing for our systems. (The Food and Drug Administration estimates that 2 to 4% of chronic NSAID users will develop upper gastrointestinal bleeding, a symptomatic ulcer, or an intestinal perforation. A recent paper from the Dennemiller Memorial Educational Foundation calculates that up to 20,000 deaths occur annually from these causes.) Besides, *any* usage of drugs—short-, medium- or long-term—hasn't been all that effective for a lot of us. Just go back and re-read some of the comments in the previous two chapters if you doubt it. On this score a survey referred to in an article in the December 1996 issue of *Reader's Digest*—"Relieving Chronic Pain Without Drugs"—found 44% of people with mild to moderate chronic pain continued to suffer while taking pain medication.

This area of unorthodox, non-traditional medicine has received various seals of approval in spite of some physicians being unwillingly dragged along. The American Medical Association (AMA), in Resolution # 514, encourages its members "to become better informed regarding alternative (complementary) medicine and to participate in appropriate studies of it." A few well regarded hospitals have begun to create alternative medical clinics in their facilities. Almost one-third of American medical schools—among them Harvard, Yale, Johns Hopkins and Georgetown Universities—now offer coursework in alternative medicine. The National Institutes of Health (NIH) has both an Office of Alternative Medicine (OAM) and an Office of Dietary Supplements (ODS). The most recent stamp of governmental approval came in October 1998, with the establishment of the National Center for Complementary and Alternative Medicine. The Center will be supporting research and disseminating information on complementary and alternative medicine to both practitioners and the public.

Recent statistics demonstrate the extent to which the public has embraced non-traditional therapies. In a late

1998 survey published in the AMA Journal, 40% of Americans were found to employ them.

Overview

There are dozens of alternative therapies which people are now using for various ailments. Some seem rather far fetched. In this chapter I've included pretty much whatever I could find which has been tried for the treatment of neuropathic pain. (The next chapter covers vitamins, herbs and other nutritional supplements, which also are considered alternative approaches to dealing with PN.) You the reader can then decide which you may wish to investigate further. My reason for such a broad coverage? What some medical professionals may regard as quackery, in fact, appears to work for some people. The bottom line with any PN treatment is whether it gives relief to the individual who's trying it.

An editorial in the August 1997 issue of *Aids Care* makes an important point:

> "We don't know the answer to that question [why AZT prevents mother-to-child transmission of HIV]. We don't know the answers to many such questions, but we do know that certain therapies work, at least in some patients, some of the time. . . . Never argue with success." [1]

---

[1] For a different point of view consider the following comment from Michael R. Clark, M.D., assistant professor of psychiatry and director of Chronic Pain Services in the Department of Psychiatry at John Hopkins:

"I'm really an advocate for a thorough evaluation. We're not against alternatives, in the sense of alternative vs. traditional medicine.

Nevertheless, to offer a little pilotage through these murky waters, the treatments in this chapter are discussed in a descending order of "apparent medical acceptance." The ranking is based solely on my own perceptions of how doctors feel about them. From what I've seen, medical judgments are usually determined in the first instance by how scientific a particular procedure seems to practitioners based on clinical reports and "the literature."[2] These judgments appear to be frequently tempered and modified by feed-back received from their patients—if the doctors have open minds.

I must say that after "Physical Therapy," discussed first, medical acceptance of these treatments seems to drop off rather sharply. Each of the treatments in the chapter has some proponents, though. In the end, as indicated before, the PNer must decide for himself or

---

After all, today's traditions are yesterday's alternatives. What made them traditions was a thorough evaluation and systematic research, just like the research Dr. Staats is doing with the snail toxin. [Author's note: This is covered in the chapter on Experimental Drugs.] When people go out and buy herbs, there's little research or data to support their effectiveness. Patients suffering from chronic pain are very vulnerable; they can be scammed very easily. I just want patients to be confident and informed consumers. Demand to know why somebody's doing something and *demand to see the data on why it works*. [emphasis supplied]"

[2] If one were to take a poll among users of these various treatments I suspect a very different ranking would emerge. For example, though doctors, who are not crazy about either, would seem to put acupuncture above magnets, most PNers appear to accept magnets more readily as you will see from their comments. Clinical trials, or the lack thereof, do not mean a lot when your feet are hurting and you're getting relief from your magnet shoe inserts—or you think you are.

herself what's worthwhile attempting, particularly when nothing tried before may have been effective.

Physical Therapy

Physical therapy involves **stretching** and **strengthening muscles** and **improving** the range of **joint motion**. Treatment options can include exercises for flexibility, strength and stability. It can be administered in a special facility with various kinds of equipment for the therapist to use with the client, or it can be accomplished in a client's home or place of business.

Advocates claim that physical therapy treatments can benefit anyone who has a **connective tissue problem**, such as muscle spasms, trauma, chronic pain, and neuromuscular conditions.

I did (partially) go through a physical therapy program myself about 18 months ago. My therapist first made a video of me walking fast on a treadmill (try that when your feet are really aching) and pronounced that I had a foot pronation problem which I knew already and was wearing orthotics because of it. Then over the course of a half dozen treatment sessions he had me go through various series of stretching exercises involving muscles in my calves, back, chest and neck, as well as the Achilles tendons.

I really felt all these exercises would probably have done me more good than they did if I had stayed with the program longer. I figured, though, once I got the hang of it I could do them at home and I stopped going back to the clinic. Probably a mistake because I gave those exercises up after a while.

In the *Chronic Pain Workbook* previously referred to, Robert W. Allen, M.D., writes:

> "In any case, physical therapy is absolutely mandatory in cases of CRPS ['complex regional pain syndrome,' a type of neuropathic pain oftentimes resulting from trauma]. Any effort you make at increasing the use of your arm or leg is beneficial. The less you move your affected arm or leg, the more likely it is that the limb will become nonfunctional. Physical therapy for CRPS often involves gentle exercises to increase flexibility as well as prevent stiff joints and osteoporosis due to lack of movement."

Whether or not a PNer goes through a formal PT program (and it may be advisable for many), I am firmly convinced that a good exercise routine—as much and of the kind that a PNer can tolerate—is really important. It will not only help your body remain healthy and preserve its strength, but also it will give you a more positive mental outlook. More on that later when we talk about exercise.

As with many of the alternative treatments mentioned in this chapter, physical therapy is often used in conjunction with other approaches to pain relief as a few of the following comments indicate.

[comments re physical therapy are not to be considered medical opinions and should not be relied upon as such—always consult your doctor:

(1) Five years ago, after receiving my diagnosis of PN I became depressed; I researched it and my depression deep-

ened. Having been healthy all my life (I'm a grandmother many times over) I felt as if life as I knew it was over for me. I was wrong. A combination of an anti-depressant (Paxil), slow progression of the disease, and **physical therapy** with a caring and knowledgeable therapist has worked magic. I tire easily, am able to manage the nerve pain and the leg muscle "knots" by working through them and feel very fortunate. There is help out there but you have to keep trying to find the people who can help. I'm still on the Paxil and have to smile to myself when I think how I resisted taking it for so very long. It was my first step toward putting myself together again and my children and grandchildren appreciate my efforts AND SO DO I. Anon

(2) I have found **physical therapy** beneficial. It has helped to improve and restore my balance. It has helped with breathing through the pain and stress related tension/pain. It has restored my ability to sit and rise from seated position without the use of pillows, chair arms or my hands. It has enabled me to walk more rapidly (this in itself helps with balance). I still walk looking down at all the cracks in the sidewalk so I don't trip and fall but I walk. It worked for me. Anon

(3) The doctor in charge of the **physical therapy** unit at the hospital recommended I try a course of PT as long as my health insurance would pay for it. He then said, "Of course it won't help your neuropathy, but it'll tone your muscles up a little." I didn't pursue it. Keith

(4) I was told by my neurologist to try [**physical therapy**] to strengthen my back. He said this might unblock nerves from my back to my feet. I tried it and it didn't seem to work. However, I may have given up too soon. If it works for anybody else, I'll go back to the grind. Robert

(5) I too was told that PT [**physical therapy**] would help, and then told it wouldn't help at all. Yes, it's very frustrat-

ing. It's bad enough we get different answers from different Dr.'s but sometimes even from the same Dr. As someone on this site said a while back, that's why they call it "Medical Practice." It's us they are practicing on. Marilyn

(6) PT [**physical therapy**] hasn't helped at all with my PN, but it has done me a world of good in strengthening muscles and restoring nerve pathways after the spinal cord injury that caused my PN in the first place. I have greatly restored function. I recommend PT to anyone who has weakened muscles for whatever reason. Robert

(7) After two sessions of acupuncture my doctor asked whether I had experienced any relief from pain—even for a little while. I told him I had not and he replied that he was sorry but he feared he could not help me. He did refer me to a nutritionist, who put me on B6, B12 and folic acid. But what really did help me was **physical therapy** with a therapist who uses the Feldenkrais method [described as a method of using slow, gentle movements "within the limits of avoiding pain"]. Anon]

Psychotherapy

According to many experts, a PNer's state of mind can have significant effects on his or her perception of pain. Psychotherapists help their patients deal with this pain in various ways including **relaxation** and **meditation training**, **biofeedback techniques** and **hypnosis**.

The philosophy common to these approaches is the belief that patients (a.k.a. clients) can do something on their own to control their pain. In other words, it returns responsibility to the individual instead of having the doctor take care of everything. People also may be required either to change their attitudes toward their pain or to realize how different forces and events have contributed to their predicament.

Quite often the following procedures (as well as others covered in this chapter) are used with other treatments at the same time. Medical professionals would tend to describe these psychotherapy procedures as "adjuvant therapies"—meaning therapies used in addition to the primary treatment—though one may sometimes wonder which should be considered primary and which adjuvant.

1. Relaxation and Meditation Training

This procedure is used to teach people to relax tense muscles and reduce anxiety. It's been demonstrated that both **physical** and **mental tension** can make any pain worse (and can even be the primary cause of pain in some cases). Alternatively, pain can often be reduced when one practices **relaxation techniques**. In fact, relaxation can act synergistically with pain medications, helping them do their job more readily and effectively.

When a person becomes tense because of pain or other stresses a reaction known as the **"stress response"** or the **"fight-or-flight response"** often occurs. This reaction causes the body to immediately release **norepinephrine** and **adrenaline** as a first-line of defense against the stress.

The theory is that if these chemicals course through the body for a lengthy period of time they will increasingly aggravate the pain already present, causing the release of yet more chemicals, and on and on. If the body, however, can be induced to relax, chemical changes such as an increased production of beneficial neurotransmitters and a reduction in the out-pouring of the stress chemicals will take place which will ultimately reduce the pain.

An excellent way to release tension and relax is by consciously **breathing deeply**. This helps immediately assure there's enough oxygen in the body for all its functions. It's been suggested by therapists that whenever someone feels sudden stress or sharp pain coming on they should immediately take five or six deep breaths. It can be done simply by closing your eyes and concentrating on inhaling slowly and deeply and then exhaling completely after each breath.

One of the great things about deep breathing as a relaxation technique is that it can be done anywhere and at almost any time. Professionals say that if one will take a few moments several times a day to do a few deep breathing exercises there will be a cumulative effect which will have a noticeable effect on stress and pain reduction by day's end.

Following is a more elaborate breathing exercise adapted by psychiatrist Dr. Karen Syrjala from *The Relaxation & Stress Reduction Workbook* by M. Davis, E. Eschelman and M. McKay (New Harbinger Publications, 1995), as set forth in her own book, *The Management of Cancer Pain* (Lea & Febiger, 1990):

"Inhale through your nose and count slowly to 4. Try to fill your lungs from the lowest part to the highest part, pushing out your abdomen, then your lower ribs, then your chest as your body fills with air. Hold your breath for 3 seconds. Exhale, and try to let air out as you let it in—from lowest to highest parts of your lungs. Repeat for 5 to 10 minutes. If you become lightheaded at any point, alternate 6 regular breaths with 6 deep breaths."

Another method of relaxation is called PMR—**progressive muscle relaxation**. The idea is to contract your muscles group by group and then release the tension slowly. For example, you might concentrate on muscles in your hands and arms first, clenching your fist as tightly as possible and feeling the tightness move up your arm to your shoulder. After holding the tension momentarily you would release your fist and let your arm go limp. Then you might start on the muscles in your feet, legs and thighs by stretching first one foot straight out as far as possible until you feel tightness creep up your leg before letting go and moving on to the other.

There are books covering PMR techniques in detail such as *The Relaxation & Stress Reduction Workbook* mentioned above.

People who undertake a regular program of practicing relaxation techniques are urged to find one that seems to work best and then stick with it until it becomes routine. A minimum of five to ten minutes a day is suggested. The point is also made that, as with any exercise, it may take time before the full benefits are felt. Some practitioners say to allow two weeks before assessing results.

Another method which works for some people is simply listening to **cassette tapes** playing soft music, or sounds of ocean waves, wind in the trees or a running brook, for example.

Meditation training tries to teach people to step back from pain which may be dominating their lives and in effect "uncouple" themselves from its perception. The idea is to make people realize thoughts and feeling about pain are quite different from the pain itself. It is very much a "mind over matter" technique. Yet it appears to work for "some people, some of the time. . . ." In fact according to one study reported in the *Reader's Digest* December 1996 article, "Relieving Chronic Pain Without Drugs," 72% of those in pain who practiced meditation felt a one third reduction in its intensity.

[comments re relaxation and meditation are not to be considered medical opinions and should not be relied upon as such—always consult your doctor:

(1) I appreciate the fact that others know what the pain and those awful electric shocks feel like. I go to many business meetings in the course of my week and feel like a fool when I jerk my legs about. **Deep breathing**, whistling and even singing (only when very alone) seem to relieve some of those little stabs. Anne

(2) The thing that has worked the best for me at night to help me go to sleep, and when I wake during the night, is to play a guided **meditation tape**. It takes your mind off your pain and because most of them are designed to relax you, I have never come to the end of the tape awake. During meditation is the only time I am without pain. I'd be pleased to give you the names of some, if you're interested. But if you go to a store, be sure it's a GUIDED meditation, not just music (although that's nice sometimes too). Some of them have guided meditation on one side and just music on the other. DON'T GIVE UP, CONCENTRATE ON WHAT YOU CAN DO, NOT ON WHAT YOU CAN'T. Velda]

2. Biofeedback

Biofeedback is a procedure in which people are taught to control their health by the use of **signals** from their own bodies. These signals can be picked up by an instrument which acts like a sixth sense and allows people to "see" or "hear" activity in their own bodies. For example, one particular device picks up signals from muscles where electrodes have been attached to the skin and activates a **beeper** or **electric light** every time the **muscles tense**. Hearing or seeing this, the subject can try to minimize the beeping or flashing by relaxing. With practice one learns how to alter the signals and keep the muscles relaxed by making internal body adjustments.

There are other ways biofeedback training might help a person regulate biological processes. For example, with the use of a **thermometer** feeding information about **hand temperatures**, a subject can often learn to change temperature at will after a few days of practice! Heart rates, blood pressure and brain activity can be monitored and controlled in the same way.

The principal difference between biofeedback and other psychotherapy procedures such as relaxation training is its employment of instruments to **relate information** back to the patient. These instruments can be as simple as the thermometer in the foregoing example or as sophisticated as an electroencephalograph which measures brain wave patterns.

Biofeedback is frequently directed to **altering usual reactions** to stress that lead to pain or disease. Experts say it can also assist in managing existing pain problems. To take one illustration, by controlling muscular contraction and spasm it is said one can learn how to keep pain from spreading to other parts of the body.

There are various chronic pain conditions which reportedly have been successfully treated by biofeedback. **Migraine** and **tension headaches** are notable examples. The *Reader's Digest* article, "Relieving Chronic Pain Without Drugs," previously referred to, mentions a study where chronic headache sufferers who completed 6 to 20 biofeedback sessions reduced their use of pain medications by 56% and headache related doctor visits by an average of 75%.

The *UC Berkeley Wellness Letter* (April 1997) reported that biofeedback training has also been used to treat musculoskeletal disorders and many other problems. The article pointed out, however, that not all types of pain respond to the reduction of muscle tension—a goal of biofeedback training.

Biofeedback is often used in conjunction with relaxation exercises. Researchers have discovered that those who benefit the most from this procedure have already trained themselves to relax and modify their behavior. (Interestingly, though, some people who generally feel uncomfortable with relaxation techniques may trust biofeedback because it seems more scientific to them.) Biofeedback trainers say that ultimately the real success of the procedure depends on the **motivation** of the person involved.

The Association for Applied Psychophysiology and

Biofeedback has a good deal of helpful information which they will make available to you without charge, including a list of their publications. They suggest you send a stamped return envelope for this purpose to their offices at Suite 304, 10200 W. 44th Ave., Wheat Ridge, CO 80033.

[comments re biofeedback are not to be considered medical opinions and should not be relied upon as such—always consult your doctor:

(1) **Biofeedback** can be a real help in controlling PN pain when used in conjunction with exercise, vitamins, diet, rest, etc. I use it daily to control my PN pain. I choose not to use the traditional pain medications mainly because I have a low tolerance for the medications and the side effects really affect my quality of life. My husband is a Certified Biofeedback Therapist (now retired) who was in private practice in a Pain Clinic. His patients were chronic pain sufferers (migraine, etc.) There is a good success rate with migraine headache sufferers, but I don't think there is much data on the success of PN pain patients and biofeedback. Your success will depend on how hard you are willing to work at it. It is not a miracle cure. Don't expect to do three sessions and stop. It is an on-going process. I have my own therapist here at home, so I have an advantage but I know it works. If nothing else you will be able to see how your mind controls your body and the pain. One thing I do suggest is to make sure you are seeing a Certified Biofeedback Therapist . . . one who has a certification from an accredited biofeedback training facility AND has experience with chronic pain patients. Some psychologists have no training and little chronic pain experience and are doing biofeedback therapy. Make sure your therapist has the right credentials. You'll get more out of the sessions

with a therapist properly trained. Good luck with your sessions. It will work if you want it to!! Dottie

(2) Following an auto accident in 1978 I could not shake the pain for two years. I could not take pain killers because at the time I was traveling the Freeways of LA for a living. I tried **Bio-feedback** for awhile, and while hooked to the machine I could cause it to be silent, showing that I was affecting my state of relaxation. During that brief period I was pain free . . . but an hour later the pain was very much evident. If I had stayed with the program I might have had greater success but I didn't want to buy the machine. Woody]

3. Self Hypnosis

Hypnosis is an induced **subconscious state**, much like a trance, which some proponents claim can be useful therapeutically. The idea is that when a person enters this state and tunes out the surrounding environment, he or she is more susceptible to **suggestions**.

The procedure has been demonstrated to be helpful in pain relief. For example researchers at the Fred Hutchinson Cancer Research Center in Seattle, in a test involving 45 patients undergoing bone marrow transplants, determined that hypnosis used with pain medication was more effective than pain medication alone.

In **self hypnosis** the suggestions are given by the subject directly to his or her own subconscious mind without the intervention of a hypnotist. Some of the ways this may be done are covered in *Hypnosis for Change* by J. Hadley and C. Staudacher (Ballantine Books, 1987) and *Self-Hypnosis: The Complete Manual for Health and Self-Change* (Souvenir, 1993).

Practitioners say a key to self hypnosis is for the subject to learn to become **totally relaxed** and let go completely so that the subconscious takes charge. Once a hypnotic trance is reached with the subconscious in control the subject might then listen to **pre-recorded tapes** (which perhaps have been made in his or her own voice) to help achieve a pre-determined purpose.

Dr. Joseph Barber, an eminent psychotherapist, has outlined several techniques for pain relief while in a self-induced hypnotic trance. These include imagining you're gradually turning down the volume on your pain until it disappears; substituting another kind of sensation—such as a feeling of being hot or cold—for the pain sensation; or relocating your pain to some other place in your body where it's "out of the way" and not interfering with any of your activities. Once you've convinced your "inner self" that one of these objectives has been accomplished the inner self is instructed to maintain the desired state into the future.

Who knows, self hypnosis may work for any PNer in helping relieve pain. For some it could certainly be worth a try (though I have to frankly add, not for me).

4. Prayer

I'm not sure this sub-section belongs under "Psychotherapy." Perhaps it should stand on its own. There is no doubt, though, that many PNers receive **solace** from **prayer** and **going to church or temple**, consequently improving their mental states, giving them peace and better enabling them to deal with their affliction. PNers are not alone in benefiting from such activities.

In the lead article in the October 1998 issue of *Reader's Digest*, "Faith Can Heal," the author cites a couple of interesting studies. In one, 455 elderly hospital patients who attended church more than once a week were found to average 4 days in the hospital versus 10 to 12 days for those who rarely or never attended church. A Yale University study of 2812 elderly people determined that those who often or altogether skipped church had nearly twice the stroke rate of weekly churchgoers.

An article in the September 24, 1998, edition of *The Canadian Press*, describes another study of 4000 people aged 65 and older. It found those who participated in religious activities were 40% less likely to have high blood pressure than those without a spiritual life. The article also claims that research has shown that "religious" people are less depressed and have better immune systems.

Skeptics might argue that people in these groups might well have shared other characteristics which were more relevant to their health; for example, that perhaps the churchgoers smoked and drank alcoholic beverages less than those in the control groups. However, a study similar to those above and funded by the National Institutes of Health claimed to have made statistical adjustments for these factors in concluding prayer was beneficial to the participants' health. (The study involved 2000 older adults over a six-year period and determined that those who attended religious services at least once a week and prayed at least once a day were 40% less likely to have high blood pressure than those who performed such activities less frequently.)

As an example of the inroads "faith healing" is making in medicine, the author of the *Digest* article just mentioned said that all American residency programs for new psychiatrists are now required to address religious and spiritual issues. He also noted that a faith-and-medicine course has been taught for three years at John Hopkins School of Medicine.

Incidentally, the November 1998 issue of *The Johns Hopkins Newsletter* has an article, "Can Religion Be Good Medicine?" which makes the interesting point that religion seems to act as a **buffer** against spiritual and physical pain. The authors mention a study in which 40% of 542 hospitalized patients said their religious faith was the most important factor in coping with their illnesses.

The authors of the article contend the principal scientific basis for how praying influences health is that it **reduces stress**, causing the body's adrenal glands to become less active in releasing the chemicals that tend to raise heart rates and blood pressures. This is, of course, much the same as the reasoning behind relaxation and meditation training.

Beyond the fact that prayer demonstrably provides **"natural"** therapeutic benefits, many will point out that on occasion a seeming **supernatural outcome** follows prayer. Certainly if a healing takes place in *another* person for whom prayer has been given (intercessory prayer), one can't say it is due to any therapeutic benefit.

Some will claim in these situations God must have directly intervened to produce the result—just as He was asked to do. Who really knows? After all, medical literature is filled with instances where miraculous cures have occurred following prayer—cures which cannot be explained by conventional wisdom.

Hyperbaric Oxygen Therapy

Hyperbaric oxygen therapy is a medical treatment by which oxygen is administered at greater than normal pressure to patients. It has long been used to treat carbon monoxide poisoning as well as burns and open wounds. Recently, usage has been extended to a broad list of medical problems—from spinal cord injuries to secondary infections associated with AIDS.

A patient undertaking hyperbaric oxygen therapy goes into a **special chamber** resembling a one-person submarine. (If you have claustrophobia like my wife, bless her, forget it.) **Pure oxygen** is then pumped in under pressure, resulting in a final oxygen concentration 10 to 15 times that of outside air. The pressure is said to force the oxygen into body tissues, supposedly restoring circulation where blood flow had been previously reduced or restricted.

Several years ago a study reported by SEARCH Alliance was undertaken to assess the efficacy of the treatment for peripheral neuropathy in HIV patients. Although nerve conduction tests did not show any objective benefit for the ten patients who underwent the test, seven reported subjectively that the numbness and lethargy which they had felt before was diminished.

Even if it is someday demonstrated to be more beneficial than now thought for PNers, there are two possible strikes against hyperbaric oxygen therapy: its high cost and the relative inaccessibility of treatment centers. Almost all of the 300 or so hyperbaric oxygen chambers in the U.S. are located in hospitals or other institutions.

There is at least one company offering something called "**aerobic oxygen**." According to Good For You Canada Corporation (how about that for an uplifting name), its aerobic product is stabilized oxygen in a non-toxic liquid form. The result, according to Good For You, is that more oxygen is introduced into the blood stream than through normal breathing processes.

The company is rather coy in talking about the product's benefits. They say in their sales literature, when answering the hypothetical question of what can be expected from using it: "Everyone is different, and therefore no one can say what the product can do for you. Look at the qualities of oxygen and judge for yourself—you will never know until you try it!"

Another oxygen-based therapy reportedly used by a few practitioners involves **ozone**. Whereas most oxygen molecules in the atmosphere have two atoms of that element (O_2), ozone has three (O_3). Ordinarily this reactive form of oxygen is quite toxic and creates free radicals which are the very targets of antioxidant therapies. When it is properly administered under controlled conditions, however, ozone supposedly can produce beneficial effects such as enhancing the body's immune system. In these procedures ozone is either injected directly into the skin or muscle, or is infused into blood which has been withdrawn from a patient and then pumped back in. The latter process is known as **autohemotherapy**.[3]

Acupuncture

A good deal of what is labeled alternative medicine comes from other cultures or from ancient traditions. **Acupuncture** is a prime example. It has been documented as being in use in ancient China as early as 2697 B.C.[4]

In spite of countless generations of users in the Far

---

[3] A doctor reviewing a draft of this book warned of the potentially toxic nature of these procedures. He suggested I advise readers I am not recommending them as suitable treatment therapies. Let me say it again: I am NOT recommending *any* therapy or procedure mentioned in this book. My role is simply to bring information to your and your doctor's attention. Nuff said?

[4] Not singling out acupuncture particularly, I thought the following comment on whether a therapy is somehow proven valid by long use was interesting, even if you don't accept its point of view:

"This ploy [stating that a particular therapy has been "time tested"] suggests that the length of time a remedy has been used is a measure of its effectiveness. Its promoters imply that if the remedy didn't work, it wouldn't remain available. Some promoters claim (sometimes truthfully, sometimes not) that their methods have been handed down from generation to generation, are steeped in folk wisdom, were derived from ancient writings, or the like. The falsity of this ploy is easily seen by noting that astrology has survived for thousands of years with no reliable evidence of any validity." From the *Quackwalk Home Page*, by Drs. Stephen Barrett and Victor Herbert.

East and in other parts of the world, acupuncture was slow to gain acceptance in this country. It got its big push here in 1972 when famed journalist James Reston underwent an emergency appendectomy during a trip to China. He wrote a front-page story for *The New York Times* reporting how it relieved his postoperative pain. Following that article demand for the technique took off in the United States.

The classical Chinese theory behind acupuncture bears little resemblance to Western medical thinking, as is true with many alternative therapies with a Far Eastern genesis. Under the Chinese theory, the important factor in maintaining pain-free health is assuring that our body energy, called **qi**, is unimpeded and flows smoothly. According to this view, channels of qi, called **meridians**, run in ordered patterns throughout the body. (These channels or patterns have little correspondence to nerve trunks in our nervous systems.) Obstructions in the meridians cause deficiencies of energy, blood and nerve pulses, eventually leading to disease. Specific points along meridians are given names pertaining to, for example, a hand or a foot. The idea is that thin **stainless steel needles** properly placed at these points, which are sometimes twirled and to which heat or an electric current are sometimes supplied, unblock the channels. According to this theory, the regular flow of qi to a particular body part is reestablished, promoting health and relieving pain.

The Western explanation is that acupuncture needles **stimulate nerves** and cause certain **chemicals** (for example endorphins, a naturally occurring pain killer in the body) to be **released** in the muscles, spinal cord and brain. Under this view, these chemicals either will change the experience of pain or will trigger the release of other chemicals and hormones which influence the body's own regulating system.

The therapy seems to be gaining legitimacy regardless of the rationale adopted. Although the American Medical Association doesn't officially sanction acupuncture, it's reported that 2000 of this country's 12,000 acupuncturists are M.D.s. The National Institutes of Health in November 1997, in fact, put its imprimatur on the treatment, stating there is "clear evidence" that it can help ease post-operative nausea as well as nausea caused by chemotherapy and pregnancy. In the April 1, 1998, issue of the prestigious journal, *Nature*, the following comment was made:

> "Research has shown that acupuncture has relieved pain in 70 per cent of [people] who have sought treatment. Clinical trials show acupuncture is successful in treating osteoarthritis of the knee, tennis elbow, headaches, facial and back pain. In the United States alone, one million people use acupuncture each year."

The World Health Organization has gone on record as stating that several groups of diseases, *including peripheral neuropathy*, respond well to acupuncture treatment. Dr. Lee Nauss, an anesthesiologist at the prestigious Mayo Pain Clinic, reports that Mayo uses acupuncture if patients don't respond to the more traditional types of treatments such as medications and nerve blocks.

There have been a few clinical studies concerning acupuncture's efficacy in providing PN pain relief and they seem to go in all directions. At a conference held in Paris in 1990, a French acupuncturist reported that among 31 subjects with HIV-related peripheral neuropathy who underwent one to three acupuncture treatments a week, 12 had their pain completely alleviated and 11 others experienced relief of most of their symptoms. In a later study at Boston University School of Medicine (reported in the August 1997 issue of *Aids Care*) researchers using acupuncture reported "significantly improved sensations" among 7 out of 26 participants who had HIV-related peripheral neuropathies.

A markedly different result was reported from a much larger study completed in late 1997 under a rigorous National Institute of Allergy and Infectious Disease (NIAID) protocol. In evaluating separately and together acupuncture and amitriptyline for the relief of PN pain for HIV-infected patients, the study concluded that "neither this standardized acupuncture regimen nor amitriptyline was effective in relieving pain."

A still later study performed at the Department of Medicine, Manchester Royal Infirmary, University of Manchester, U. K. (reported in the February 1998 issue of *Diabetes Research and Clinical Practice*), considered acupuncture for the treatment of chronic peripheral *diabetic* neuropathy.[5] There among 46 patients who were

---

[5] Most of the clinical studies concerning peripheral neuropathies are limited to either HIV or diabetic victims for the simple reason that that's where the research money is, in this country and elsewhere, either from pharmaceutical companies or from government funding.

treated with acupuncture 29 already were on "standard medical treatment." Patients initially received up to six courses of classical acupuncture over a period of 10 weeks, using traditional Chinese acupuncture points. Forty-four completed the study with 34 (77%) showing significant improvement in their primary and/or secondary symptoms. These were followed up for a period of 18–52 weeks with 67% said to have been able to stop or reduce their medications significantly. Seven, in fact, noted their symptoms cleared completely. The data suggested to the researchers that "acupuncture is a safe and effective therapy for the long-term management of painful diabetic neuropathy, although its mechanism of action remains speculative."

A somewhat related procedure called "**acupressure**" involves using finger pressure instead of needles at the same points or loci which acupuncturists use. The fact that the technique is non-invasive obviously appeals to many.

"**Moxibustion**" is a procedure even more distantly related to acupuncture. It involves the burning of **mugwort** over acupuncture points. According to Western thinking, if pain is being relieved it's because a counter-irritant was produced—much as if mustard plaster had been used. The Chinese would say the moxibustion (*jiu fa*) caused energy to be propelled into the body from outside and that it was fed it into a weak and deficient system. There does seem to be something demonstrably efficacious about the procedure in at least one situation: a recent study was conducted of 260 pregnant Chinese women whose babies were still in the breech after 33 weeks. Of these, seventy five percent who received moxibustion treatments eventually had normal head-first deliveries. Only 48 % of those in the group who did not receive treatments were able to deliver their babies normally.

Another Chinese (and Indian) procedure is "**cupping**," in which heated cups are placed on the skin where small punctures have been made. A suction force is elicited which is thought to boost circulation and generally improve health.

I have tried both regular acupuncture—with wired needles—and "**French acupuncture**," both without much success. The latter is a branch of a rather esoteric procedure called **auriculotherapy** which matches specific acupuncture sites in the ear with corresponding parts of the body. Electric probes are used in it for diagnostic as well as therapeutic purposes. (Because of her dialect—I'm not very good on the receiving end of dialects—I couldn't understand whether the acupuncturist who stuck probes in my ears using the French method was diagnosing or treating me or both. I never did find out and since I didn't get anything out of it anyway I jumped off the table and left as soon as the current was turned off.)

Regardless of my own experience, if acupuncture helps anyone (as it seemingly does based on the Manchester study cited above), God bless them and God bless acupuncture.

[comments re acupuncture are not to be considered medical opinions and should not be relied upon as such—always consult your doctor:

(1) My husband, Dave, went to a Chinese M.D. here in NJ who has a good reputation for **acupuncture** help. The dr. said that if there was no improvement after four treatments, Dave should stop because that meant it wasn't going to work. Dave took his 4 treatments—no improvement—no change at all, so he quit and has not been back. Anon

(2) Yes, I tried **acupuncture**. With a Chinese practitioner. The first few treatments; nothing. Then I started getting some relief. Short lived (a matter of a day or so), but improvement. Some relief turned into more relief at about the four week mark, but then I hit a limit. For the first time I began feeling the needles, and it was extremely painful. I was forced to stop treatment. Jim

(3) I also tried **acupuncture** combined with electro-stimulation. Like Jim, at first it was painless and seemed to help me get through a particularly painful period. At about the 13th time, I nearly jumped off the table when the needles were inserted. I asked if the acupuncturist was using a larger needle (no). I was able to tolerate a much lower electro-stim. And I didn't return for additional treatments. Marjorie

(4) I have several friends who are **acupuncturists**. One is a Chinese man with a MD degree from Johns Hopkins (I believe) and is the founder and head of the Acupuncture College of the Southwest. He told me that acupuncture does not help the kind of PN that I have. I took his word for it. Jim P.

(5) I just had my first **acupuncture** treatment today. It did help pain as long as needles were in. But I didn't make it out of the office before it was coming back. This afternoon, I have had a huge increase in pain. Haven't been this bad in 18 months. Has anyone else experienced this? I am already dreading going back next week. Anon.

(6) I have had four treatments so far from a master **acupuncturist** (DO). They have reduced but not eliminated the pain. Yes, it does seem to wear off. He also has me on Chinese herbs to promote nerve healing. He feels it will take about 4 months on the herbs. Nice side effect is I am slowly loosing weight!! Just a little each week—but that is OK. He also recommends chelation treatments. I can't afford them unless my insurance will pay. I'm trying to research this for others' experiences. So far only replies have been somewhat positive. I'm not sure about it yet. If anyone has experiences please let me know. Bob

(7) Yes, I have tried **acupuncture**. The first time the needles were put in my lower back. I had four sessions, one a week. This doctor said you have to give it at least four times to see if it was going to work. After the second treatment I could feel my feet. It was a miracle, but it only lasted a few days and it never happened again. The second time I did acupuncture with a different doctor, he put the needles up and down my legs then attached leads to the needles that transmitted electrical stimulation. This treatment lasted about 30 minutes. I did this once a week for about 3 months. No change. He also put them in my back with the electrical stimulation. Doc finally said he felt this was not going to benefit me so there was no sense continuing. At least he was honest. Neither treatment really hurt just sometimes a little uncomfortable but when you are desperate, I've tried several things with no success. HUGS sometimes work the best!!!! Mary Jane

(8) I too have been suffering with lower back pain which sometimes involves my sciatica and sometimes just hurts—it changes from the middle to side to side at will. I never associated it with PN. I've been going to an acupuncturist for it. I also have a slight herniated disc which I've blamed. Last week she gave me a DEEP **acupressure**

massage, and I thought she was killing me, but I think it helped. I'll keep you up to date on this. Velda

(9) A friend recommended a Chinese doctor in my area who is considered a physical therapist, and does **acupressure**. I went to him one time, because I have alot of pain with PN in my hands and feet, from Carpal tunnel, and herniated disc. It was very interesting, and he worked on my arms, shoulders and hands (mostly on the left side which is worse). I was very tender in the areas where he massaged. Everytime I blurted out an "ow," he knew where to massage. The Chinese believe in working on the tendons, which are connected to the nerves and muscles. He said he believed he could help me, and if it did not he would not ask me for a penny! He believes it will not be alot of sessions . . . like Chiropractors do, I have already been down that road. He does not like them, and says most don't know what they are doing. He has a few clients that are rich, and fly him to where they are and work on them. He got all his techniques from his mother, who is now deceased. He also has a regimine of exercises that are very important for improvement, and are based on what your condition is. I am having my second appointment tomorrow, and am going to ask him to work on my feet, because the pain from the disc produces pain in my hands, and I already have CT, so they are always in pain. I think I can stand my hands more than my feet. I will keep you informed of my progress if you would like me to. Good luck! P.S. He may do acupuncture also, but I think he specializes more in acupressure, and I guess I will find out more on my second visit. Suellen]

Touch (and Near Touch) Therapies

The therapies covered in this section involve using hands or devices to **stimulate nerves** and **muscles** and/or to **release tensions** and the body's "natural life forces." The most familiar example is the **massage**, certainly a procedure with a long history similar to acupuncture's. (In fact in the tomb of Ankh-mahor, said to date back to 2200 B.C., there is a depiction of an Egyptian priest giving a man a foot massage—perhaps one of our earliest PNers.)

1. Basic and Other Massages

Enhanced blood flow is the direct effect of applying manual pressure in a rhythmic way to different parts of the body. The resulting improvement in circulation is said to increase the **oxygen capacity** of blood by 10 to 15 per cent and assist in the removal of wastes and toxins.

Massaging also allows **muscular systems** to **relax**, thereby reducing stress. Further, the technique reportedly enables the brain to produce more pain killing **endorphins**. Another claimed effect is that massaging causes **neurons** where the massaging is being performed to "**fire up**." Once chemical signals are "fired" along nerve pathways the original pain signals are overtaken and temporarily dulled.

Massage pressure can be applied with the entire hand, the heel of the hand, the fingertips or knuckles. Supposedly the one giving the massage can feel around where pain appears to be emanating to locate "**trigger points**." Pressure can then be concentrated at these points. It is claimed pain is often relieved for several minutes and sometimes for several hours after the pressure is released.

Occasionally, **creams** or **ointments** are used with the massaging. In addition to capsaicin preparations such as Zostrix previously discussed, these can include **menthol preparations** such as Ben-Gay, Icy Hot, Mineral Ice, and Heet. When rubbed into the skin, they help to further increase blood circulation and produce a warm (sometimes cool) soothing feeling which can last for several hours.

Sometimes **vibrators** are employed in place of hands to produce a massaging effect. I used an electric foot vibrator for years when my pain really got bad with satisfactory (but only temporary) results. At least I could more blissfully read or watch TV and not think about my feet while the thing was running.[6] There are also **wooden** "massagers," really just half inch or so wooden wheels rotating on a small rod, that sell for under $10. I tried one of these on the soles of my feet a couple of times but never could figure out what it was supposed to be doing.

There are different kinds of massages. The **"Swedish"** is the one most often practiced in the West. In addition to

---

[6] There is a company in Israel, Yonitech Laboratories, Ltd., which supposedly is developing a massage unit to be used specifically for treating foot disorders of the PN type. Deep massage to the feet is said to be provided with revolving conic massage elements. The developer claims it uniquely activates neurological systems in the body. A representative of the company told me some while ago that clinical trials "with very positive results" have been performed and promised to have them sent to me. I am still waiting.

pressure the practitioner uses long gliding strokes as well as kneading and pummeling different areas of the body. This is the type which seems closest to that advocated for peripheral neuropathy therapy by Drs. G. Keith Stillwell and Gudni Thorsteinsson in their paper, "Rehabilitation Procedures" (appearing in the treatise, *Peripheral Neuropathy*, Dyck & Thomas, W. B. Saunders, 1993). The authors there suggest a "sedative" approach be used with gentle stroking and mild kneading rather than chopping and hacking motions.

Another type is called "**Shiatsu**." This is a technique said to have been initially developed by Japanese monks. Like acupuncture, it seeks to unblock channels (meridians) of energy (qi) flowing through our bodies. Although it comes from the Japanese words meaning finger—"shi"—and pressure—"atsu," the technique involves a wrestler's entire bag of moves such as shaking, grasping, patting, lifting, pinching, rolling and punching, all in addition to just applying pressure. Shiatsu is said to require a rapport to be developed between the practitioner and the client (difficult I would think when you're being beaten up like that) so that the latter's "own self healing powers are awakened."

Myotherapy is still another massage technique said to be effective for relieving pain, stiffness and other conditions of muscular origin. Myotherapists apply gentle pressure to the muscles using their thumbs, knuckles, and elbows. As each muscle relaxes, it is gently stretched to return it to its full resting strength. Most patients are said to report good results even with long-standing conditions.

Somewhat similar to myotherapy, there are also "**my-ofascial**" (sometimes referred to as "trigger point") massages involving the application of stretching techniques and gentle pressures to the body's muscles and supportive connective tissues (fascia) at precisely defined points. A procedure often used with myofascial massages is called "**touch and spray**." Here a solution of ethyl chloride is sprayed over the muscle being stretched. This causes a localized anesthesia effect and is said to permit the return of painless function more readily.

A technique related to myofascial massages called "**rolfing**" involves deep massaging of muscle connective tissues. According to practitioners, this allows the body "to move more freely."

There isn't much clinical evidence on how any of these massaging techniques help alleviate pain—neuropathic or any other kind. Dr. William Collinge reports briefly in an article, "Scientific Support for Massage and Bodywork," excerpted from *The American Holistic Association's Complete Guide to Alternative Medicine,* that in a study of various types of massage in 52 patients with traumatically induced spinal pain, there were "significant reductions in acute and chronic pain and increased muscle flexibility and tone." The article also mentions another study which was said to demonstrate a theory mentioned above—namely that massaging enhances the body's ability to control pain by stimulating the brain to produce endorphins.

Of course I imagine all of us with sensory neuropathies have at times massaged our own feet when they were numb and aching (no inconsistency between these two symptoms for us) or rubbed our hands together to get rid of tingling sensations. And we didn't need to look at a scientific study before we did so!

[comments re massages are not to be considered medical opinions and should not be relied upon as such—always consult your doctor:

(1) I have purchased two **massagers**. First is a back massaging pad. It is the vibration type rather than the kneading, shiatzu type. I keep it at the lower end of my bed and put my legs & feet on it to go to sleep (it has an automatic shutoff after 15 minutes). It really helps for the short term. The second massager is the vibration type as well, but it is a foot massager. It has many hard, immobile knobs across the top with the infrared heat in the middle. I keep this one under my desk at work. When pain gets particularly bad during the day, I have it right there. Runs very quietly. They can be purchased at various drugstores and discount chains such as Walmart. They really do help me but as I said it is short term. Their usage is particularly helpful when the need of instant (can't wait for the med to take affect) pain relief. Janet

(2) Try **massage** . . . at one point I was massaging my husband's legs a LOT [for diabetic neuropathic pain] . . . and it did help. Anon

(3) I have neuropathy in both legs and recently had swelling in feet and ankles. Tried just about everything (neurontin, supplements, epidural) with a 35% success rate with the epidural. Left with nothing more than hope, I had a deep-tissue **massage** on my leg. It reduced not only the swelling, but some of the remaining pain. By using massage, the therapist indicated it would increase the

blood supply to the area. It felt good enough to the point where I intend to continue with it. Anon]

2. Reflexology

Reflexology is a massage-like technique aimed specifically at the hands and feet. Somewhat as in acupuncture theory, it is thought there are zones in these extremities—**"reflex" areas**—which respond to stimulus. The procedure involves using thumbs and fingers to apply pressure to these zones. Practitioners claim **stress** is thereby reduced and that other **physiological changes** take place in the body which are beneficial.

Similarly to the techniques discussed above, a principal objective of reflexology is getting blood to flow more freely as a result of **stress reduction**. This in turn is supposed to lead to oxygen being carried to where it's needed and toxins and waste products removed. Other objectives are **increasing energy levels** and **restoring body balance**.

I've tried reflexology in addition to the two acupuncture procedures and magnet insertions I mention later. A reflexologist in Del Mar, California, spent about 40 minutes kneading my feet while we were chatting about how Southern California weather compares with Texas weather in August. (Mutual agreement—no comparison.) Afterwards my feet felt great—for all of 15 minutes. She told me it might take several sessions to get more lasting results. I said vaguely I might make another appointment but never did.

3. Reiki; Qigong; Therapeutic Touch

We're swimming even further from the mainstream here but each of these procedures have their proponents for pain reduction. Common elements among them are that the practitioner does not actually *massage* the body even though hands are sometimes a part of the process, and each is said to help manipulate the body's energy field.

(a) Reiki is a so-called natural healing procedure which originated in Tibet 2500 years ago and was redis-covered in Japan in the late 1800s. It is based on the be-lief that living things share **life energy**. In fact the term itself means "universal life energy." In a reiki healing session, the practitioner places his or her hands on the patient's body at one of 12 energy centers called "**chakras**." According to proponents, the patient almost always feels energy then begin to flow, often into places remote from the point at which hands have been placed. Reiki is said to "know" where it is needed and flows to the point where it can do the most good. A reiki treatment is supposed to leave the patient calm and relaxed.

(b) Qigong, a pillar of Chinese medicine, has been said to be the cultivation and refinement through prac-tice of one's **vitality** or **life force**. From a Western point of view, as with magnet therapy (discussed later), mas-saging, and reflexology, qigong is said to increase deliv-ery of oxygen to places where it's needed and to remove toxins and waste products. It's also said to affect the chemistry of the nervous system and brain. From the

Chinese perspective, it acts mainly to balance and augment natural healing resources.

Since it can be self-administered, millions of people in China individually or in groups are said to use the technique every day. Qigong exercises involve combinations of concentrated, controlled breathing with simple repetitive movements. When combined with the more active motions of Chinese martial arts it becomes **tai chi**, an excellent general exercise technique, discussed in more depth later.

So-called external qigong requires the services of an experienced practitioner who does a **non-touch** energy assessment first. The practitioner is then said to be able to project or transfer qi in a treatment mode directly to the patient for pain relief and other purposes, sometimes with his hands extended toward the patient from a distance.

(c) "**Therapeutic touch**" (TT), in spite of its name, doesn't require the therapist to actually touch the patient either. Rather the therapist's hands hover several inches over the body sensing the "**energy field pattern**" and then redirects energy into "depleted areas." Many patients are said to be able to feel the energy moving through their bodies during a therapeutic touch session. One of the explanations given by those who would rationalize this procedure is that it's based on quantum field and relativity theories. (Honestly, I didn't make that up.)

In a 1986 study by E. Keller and V. M. Bzdek (reported in the January 1996 issue of *Canadian Nurse*) the procedure was used on 60 volunteers with tension headaches.

According to the investigators, the 60 were divided into two groups, one receiving five-minute therapeutic touch interventions or treatments and the other mimicked treatments. Pain "scores" were said to have dropped an average of 70% in the group getting the actual therapy versus 37% in the other.

A 1998 study reported in the April 1st issue of *JAMA* (*The Journal Of the American Medical Association*), however, dealt a harsh blow to TT. Twenty one subjects, who were *practitioners* of the procedure, were tested under blinded conditions. They each were asked whether an investigator's unseen hand, which was hovering over their outstretched hands, was over their right hand or over their left. Pure chance, of course, would have yielded the correct answer 50% of the time. Yet they only guessed correctly in 123 of 280 trials, a 44% success rate! (The Editor of *JAMA*, in a concluding note, said the study proved that the "human energy field"—the theoretical basis for TT—simply does not exist.)

Magnets

Similarly to acupuncture, reiki and qigong, **magnetic therapy** has been used for many centuries in Eastern cultures for the treatment of pain and healing. And as with those procedures, classical-minded practitioners claim magnetic therapy achieves its benefits by re-establishing order in the energy system.

English physicians wrote about the effects of biomagnetics several hundred years ago. Later, magnetism was promoted in this country as a panacea for almost everything. In 1899 the Shimer-Gray Institute of Magnetic Healing advertised it could cure "paralysis, constipation, consumption, pleurisy, dysentery, rheumatism, piles, asthma and all female diseases," as well as "liquor, tobacco and morphine habits."

Pooh-poohed for most of the 20th century as a step just above snake oil in the therapy ladder, some practitioners have since come to believe in its benefits. For example, Dr. Paul J. Rosch, clinical professor of medicine and psychiatry at the New York Medical College and president of the American Institute of Stress, writing in the May 21st, 1998, issue of the *Medical Tribune*, said: "I believe electromagnetic field therapy will become an increasingly important component of 21st century medicine that could replace certain drugs." Some have gone much further. Ken Wiancko, M.D., wrote in the April 1995 issue of *Health Naturally*: "In a search for a universal cure-all, none fits the description nearly as well as magnetic energy therapy. The application of magnets provides proven pain relief in seven out of ten users, as good as or better than orthodox medicine."

Certainly the public has demonstrated enthusiasm for magnet therapy. It's now one of the leaders in alternative medicine usage. Today there are dozens of manufacturers of magnets sold in various forms for health and pain relief—in belts, shoe inserts, wrist bands, body patches, even in bed mattress pads. A number of golfers and other sports personalities now strap magnets on, and many of these have given glowing testimonials concerning magnets' ability to relieve pain and stiffness.

At least one obstacle preventing wider adoption by the medical profession is the fact that testing and validation of magnets' effects by manufacturers, or anybody else for that matter, is almost non-existent.

The one clinical study most often cited was performed in 1997 at Baylor University. There in a double-blind procedure 50 post-polio patients who were experiencing arthritic and muscle pains were randomly given active magnets and placebo "magnets." Seventy six percent of those who had active magnets reported a decrease in pain compared with only 19% with placebos.[7] A larger investigation is now taking place at the University of Virginia involving up to 105 volunteers with fibromyalgia— a painful muscle condition.

Some practitioners say many more studies must be made. Dr. Lauro S. Halstead at the National Rehabilitation Hospital in Washington D.C., asserts answers are needed concerning the appropriate strength of therapeutic magnets in various situations (those commonly used have a gauss strength anywhere from 300 to 700), the duration of pain relief [8] and the effects of constant usage.

---

[7] In a Letter to the Editor published in the April 1998 issue of *Archives of Physical Medicine and Rehabilitation* (p. 469), Dr. Michael I. Weintraub at the Department of Neurology, New York Medical Center in Briarcliff, New York, took issue with the Baylor study, challenging both its methodology and the parameters used to measure pain reduction.

[8] Several manufacturers subtly imply there is residual pain-relief following usage which may last for some period of time. Maybe yes, maybe no. It's not been proven. The following disclaimer from one

A few of those who believe they do work and attempt a scientific explanation for magnetics' modus operandi say it's based on the **biological effects** of magnetic fields on the living organism. The field produced from permanent magnets supposedly penetrates deeply into the skin, tissue and bones. The theory goes that the magnets generate heat, expand blood vessels and increase blood flow, bringing oxygen and nutrients to the affected area and reducing toxins. There is also speculation that stimulation by magnets at certain pain sites releases endorphins, the body's natural pain fighters and possibly the brain chemical serotonin, which enhances body relaxation. Another theory is that magnets create a field altering how pain signals are sent along the nervous system.

In spite of these hypotheses, it's not been demonstrated how magnets really deal with *neuropathic* pain (or as some would say, if at all). The principal investigator of the Baylor study, Dr. Carlos Valbona, admits he himself does not know why they benefited some in the study and not others.

The editors of the *UC Berkeley Wellness Letter*, to take one well-respected group, are more than a little cynical about all of this. They wrote in their March 1997 issue

---

maker—Magna Pak—shows they're taking no chances of being misinterpreted: "No claim is made that magnets provide a cure. Magnetic therapy products are specifically designed to increase blood circulation. If a particular condition can be helped by this increase in circulation, and the devices are properly placed, improvement should take place. *When the device is removed, the influence and the effect it has ends.* [emphasis supplied]" Clearly the lawyers are on top of the situation here.

that most therapeutic claims for magnets are "wishful thinking or outright nonsense." They continue:

> "The simple magnetic devices being sold (via mail order or 'multi-level' distributors who sell to friends and family) exert energy fields too weak to have any significant physiological effect. Thus any reported therapeutic benefits may be due to a placebo effect (or to the symptoms simply resolving themselves). That may be okay with you—if you don't mind paying $50 to $500 for a useless magnetic device. But it should not take the place of proper medical care for a serious underlying disease."

Is this a valid rejection? In any event perhaps we are left again with the premise that "whatever works. . . . " Whether or not there is a convincing scientific explanation of magnets' efficacy, they *do* appear to work for many if the comments below are good markers.[9] Before coming to those, however, a new approach in magnetic therapy should first be mentioned.

Holcomb HealthCare Services in Nashville, Tennessee, has developed a technology and a device it calls **Magna Bloc**, said to be directed specifically to the treatment of neuropathic pain. The company was founded by Dr. Robert Holcomb who holds a faculty position in the Department of Neurology at Vanderbilt University. Much of the company's investigative work, in fact, is re-

---

[9] I must say they didn't do anything more for me than acupuncture did. But as I write this and re-read all the positive comments, I've decided to slip a pair of magnetic inserts that I bought last year back into my shoes, just in case I've been missing something! (Later input, same results as before—Nada.)

portedly being done in conjunction with the Vanderbilt University Medical Center.

The Magna Bloc device is said to be a "static magnetic field generator" consisting of four magnets arranged in a square configuration with alternating polarity. The magnets are housed in a plastic case which can be attached to the skin with tape. The magnet array is said to produce a unique magnetic flux field which works by altering the wall of the nerve cell, thereby suppressing transmission of painful impulses to the brain. The company is planning to commence clinical trials preparatory to a submission to the FDA for approval of Magna Bloc as a medical treatment device.

[comments re magnets are not to be considered medical opinions and should not be relied upon as such—always consult your doctor:

(1) I want to take the time to share my new found freedom and happiness. I took a fellow BBSer's suggestion and bought **magnetic** innersoles. I bought Nikken mainly because the lady up the street was selling them and she had a pair in stock in my size. They cost $60 in the man's size large! Oh dear, my feet are big but I am almost 6' so my feet match the body. At first I was skeptical but I have been wearing them for almost three weeks with lots and lots of success. I have had PN for 8 years and have had no luck with meds and presently take none for PN. I put the innersoles in and slowly I found I could do more on my feet and I even went to a mall today. I stayed all day which I have not done since pre—PN days. I go to a local Y and I am actually enjoying my time there. I am not consumed by pain. I smile more, I look happier and I feel happier. We all know that type of pain that comes with PN where if someone walked by with a loaded gun, you want to beg them to

shoot you. You know that hair raising, nerve wrenching pain that makes life unbearable. Well the magnets for me, have given me relief. The pain is much less, not gone, but much, much less. I have a new positive attitude and refuse to let this PN take that from me. Libby

(2) I also wear the **magnets** in my shoes and wouldn't consider not using them. I tried one day without them in my shoes, that lasted about 30 minutes. I wear splints on my wrist at night with the little round magnets on the underside of my wrists. I have read where many people can not sleep because of the pain. When I go to bed I generally am pain free. My feet are extremely numb but neither my hands nor my feet hurt. If there are people out there thinking about trying them—GO FOR IT. I was a desperate woman looking for something to help even if it was short term. I have been using them for about 2 years and they just keep on giving. Now perhaps you will be able to enjoy some of life's wonderful moments. Mary Jane

(3) I saw a pain dr.-anesthesiologist first week of March and she suggested **magnet** therapy for me. I wear a magnet, sort of shaped like the heel of a man's shoe, 7" long x 5" wide. It adheres to your undies by velcro, and stays on the small of your back. It is worn 12 hrs. a day and then must be off for 12 hours a day. The brand name is Nikken. I have found it to reduce the pain in my feet noticeably. Now for the questions. No, I don't stick to the refrigerator door. Why it works. I was told it brings warmth to the area, which brings a greater blood supply, which brings more nourishment to the large number of nerves there. Judy

(4) I don't know any nice way to say this, so here goes: If a doctor makes a statement to me that "**magnets** bring warmth to the area" that doctor is incompetent, a quack, on drugs, all of the above, or worse. Beware of this guy. Pete

(5) I bought my husband **magnetic** insoles and they have helped his pain tremendously. I have ordered a magnetic

mattress pad. We are very anxious to see how it works. Doris

(6) My husband started using Nikken **magnetic** products in October and within 3 days the swelling was gone from ankles and feet, the burning was gone and the pain was gone. He still has numbness but not as bad as before. Still cannot tolerate much walking or standing, BUT he's not using a cane anymore, he's not limping and he's able to work at a very physically demanding job. He's using the mattress pad, insoles and a couple other products. Our family physician recommended trying these and they are working. Has anyone else used these? Kenneth's wife

(7) It seems I am always on the negative side. But I tried these [**magnetic**] products without any help. Jim W.

(8) I have discovered them [**magnets**]recently and think they are amazing. I don't know how they work, but they do although I'm not sure they help PN much, they do help you sleep better without meds. and work nicely on muscles aches and pains. Don't take away my Neurontin or my magnets or I will get cranky! Anon

(9) The **magnet** draws blood to the sore area, and it becomes very warm and then the pain seems to ease. I know I was taking 2 Darvocet everyday when I get home from work because my back ached so much all the time. Now I just tape the magnet on my back between my shoulders and the pain is relieved within 15–20 min. I haven't taken a pain pill since I got them. I am a real skeptic, too, as I was a surgical nurse for many years. But I think there is something happening with these magnets and I like it!! Joan]

Chelation

This is a blood therapy, controversial to say the least, sometimes used for peripheral neuropathy. It involves the **intravenous infusion** of an **organic compound** commonly referred to as **EDTA**. (You can see the reason for the acronym—the full name is ethylene diamine tetra-acetic acid.) This compound purportedly removes toxic metals such as lead, mercury and cadmium from the body. Chelation's practitioners claim (without supporting proof) that EDTA, in binding dissolved metal elements and removing them from the body, reduces abnormal production of oxygen free radical molecules which react destructively with other molecules.

The therapy requires a series of treatments (anywhere from 20 to 30) often given in a "chelation center." Each infusion, which typically takes three and a half to four hours, involves the insertion into a vein of a needle attached to a container holding about half liter of fluid in which two to three grams of EDTA have been introduced. Sometimes other substances are added such as B complex vitamins, vitamin C, magnesium and heparin (an anti-coagulant which helps prevent clotting at the injection site).

Blood and urine testing are done frequently during the course of treatment to ensure there are no kidney or liver problems. Side effects are said to be limited to possible vein irritation, headache and fatigue.

Several formulae have reportedly been developed for **oral chelation**. The claim is made that this approach does not require the same monitoring as the IV procedure and can be used as a long-term method to remove toxic metals from the blood stream. Practitioners at the Whitaker Wellness Institute disagree with the efficacy of this procedure, however. Although they maintain that IV chelation has been demonstrated to be helpful, at least for heart disease and circulatory problems, they say in their February 1997 newsletter that only five per cent of the oral EDTA is absorbed into the bloodstream, providing little or no benefit.

Although chelation is controversial, as noted, not all medical doctors dismiss its claims. One who writes a column answering submitted questions ("Dear Doctor & The Dietitian") replied that he found chelation therapy helps *most* peripheral neuropathies. The American College for Advancement in Medicine, claiming to be comprised of 750 or so licensed physicians, has written a "position paper" concerning the use of chelation for occlusive vascular and degenerative diseases associated with aging. The paper states that "chelation therapy is a valid and proper course of treatment, based upon scientific rationale, supported by many published clinical studies, and consistent with sound medical practice." Nevertheless, chelation therapy is not highly subscribed to by most practitioners today who are treating PN patients. (In fact several of the neurologists who reviewed this book think chelation is simply quackery. One saw possible value in limited cases.)

[comments re chelation are not to be considered medical opinions and should not be relied upon as such—always consult your doctor:

(1) Lee is correct when he says **chelation** is done to flush heavy metals out one's body. I've had it done several times. I went to a Dr. out in Las Vegas 2 years ago and he said the mercury in my fillings were the cause of my PN. So he recommended having fillings replaced and also chelation. It

was given in the form of an IV, and I also got some large "horse" pills that were for chelation as well. Unfortunately I didn't receive any lessening of symptoms after either the filling replacement or the chelation. Bill

(2) Janie and I have both had **chelation** therapy. For anyone who is unfamiliar with it, here is how it works: You sit in a big comfortable armchair and read a book or watch TV for about three or four hours while you get an IV of a clear liquid like colored water that contains chemicals which extract the toxins, such as plaque and heavy metals, from your arteries and tissues. The only pain or discomfort involved is in the needle prick when the IV is inserted. Then, after the IV is finished, you just go pee out the bad stuff. That's about all there is to it. It usually takes 20–30 treatments to complete the program. While we were having our treatments, we talked to some other people who had been taking them a lot longer than we have, and heard some incredible success stories. I would have been skeptical if the doctor had told me the stories, but hearing them first hand from ordinary common folks with nothing to gain from lying to us, we were very impressed. All the people told us of great success with chelation, and we heard no negative reports, except that insurance will not pay for it. As far as I know, that is the only complaint that anyone has about the chelation. I don't know why the insurance will not pay, but even if you have to pay for it out of your own pocket (around $100 per treatment), like vitamin and mineral supplements, it is a path to improving your health, and well worth the cost if it will heal you. Duncan

(3) I have experienced a 90% reduction in the neuropathy in my feet as a result of taking **chelation** treatments. From the people with neuropathy I have spoken to it appears it is caused by circulation problems. Thus that explains why the chelation treatments are so successful. I

have spoken with two people who started to experience relief after 5 treatments. In my case I started to experience relief after 9 treatments and have now taken 44 treatments and the neuropathy is now almost gone. (The angina is all gone.) Chelation with EDTA is normally administered through a 3 hour IV once a week although some physicians will administer 2 treatments per week. The treatment is seldom paid for by insurance and normally runs from $90 to $110 per treatment. Jere

(4) If anyone has been injured in a **chelation** related incident, please contact me regarding suing the doctor that charged you so much for your ineffective therapy and possible lawsuits. I am a former practitioner of chelation therapy who has proven that this treatment is worthless and does more harm than good except, of course, for those wealthy doctors who sell you the chelation package of excessive treatments, labs and special tests. These doctors make millions of dollars each year off of a scam that has no proven value. I will be willing to appear in defense of your claims if you have had no benefit or suffered injury from being led to falsely trust in chelation therapy. Please contact me at my email address. Robert]

*   *   *

There are two excellent books on alternative treatments I would certainly recommend to anyone interested in pursuing the subject: *Alternative Medicine: What Works*, by Adriane Fugh-Berman, M.D. (Williams & Wilkins, 1997) and *The Alternative Medicine Handbook*, by Barrie R. Cassileth, Ph.D. (W. W. Norton, 1998).

Chapter 6

Nutrients

Nutrients include vitamins, minerals, herbs and other supplements essential to maintaining bodily functions.[1] They usually are used by PNers as complementary to more traditional therapies.

General

Drugs and conventional medical procedures have not been very successful for many of us when used as sole treatment interventions. This is especially true when one weighs in their frequent and unwelcome side effects. Consequently, PNers have sought other approaches. So-called **natural** means of dealing with neuropathies have been favored by many, especially the use of nutrients. However, the foods we eat normally do not contain suffi-

---

[1] "Nutraceuticals" (as contrasted with "pharmaceuticals") is a term we may hear more and more in the future. It means health supplements, vitamins and other nutrients delivered to consumers through crops such as corn which sometimes have been genetically re-engineered to optimize their nutritional value.

cient amounts of these substances for **therapeutic purposes**. Thus we must add them to our diets as **supplements**.

Vitamins

Vitamins are **organic nutrients** vital for proper growth and maintenance of health. Generally, they function as **enzymes** or **catalysts** in chemical reactions which continually take place in our bodies. Vitamins are classified as being either **fat soluble**, which means they may remain in body tissues for a relatively long period of time (for example vitamins A, D, E and K), or **water soluble,** which remain in the body for only short periods before being flushed out (exemplified by vitamins B and C). These latter nutrients need to be frequently replenished.

1. Vitamin A

Beta-carotene, which is transformed into Vitamin A, is considered one of the best **antioxidants** available. Antioxidants are chemicals which kill **free radicals**. These in turn are highly reactive oxygen fragments or damaged molecules lacking one or more electrons. They are created in the body by normal chemical processes such as the conversion of food into energy. Free radicals can also be produced in dangerous amounts by irritants such as cigarette smoke, pesticides, air pollution, ultraviolet light and radiation, as well as by stress and over exercising.

Because the free-radical molecule "wants" its full com-
plement of electrons, it reacts with any molecule from
which it can take an electron. These give-away molecules
are found in certain key components such as fat, protein
or DNA. By swiping these electrons, free radicals **damage the associated cells** and cause **oxidative stress**.
According to some experts, this not infrequently leads to
peripheral neuropathy and other disorders. Antioxidants
neutralize the free radicals by giving up their electrons
easily and restoring the natural balance.

In addition to its antioxidant properties, Vitamin A
improves vision and shores up the body's immune system; it's particularly recommended for dealing with HIV
infections. Moreover it is said to fight skin disorders and
skin aging.

The **RDA** ("Recommended Daily Dietary Allowance")
for vitamin A is 5,000 IUs. Established years ago and re-
flecting views of the amounts considered adequate to
meet the *ordinary* needs of healthy individuals, many
professionals think RDAs usually fall short of what may
be necessary to keep one in optimum health, let alone
providing what many doctors think may be required to
treat a special condition such as peripheral neuropathy.
Some practitioners, for example, suggest taking from
10,000 up to 50,000 IUs daily for therapeutic purposes.
(However, it's acknowledged that at these higher levels
vitamin A should be taken under a doctor's supervision.)

At the time this was written the National Academy of
Sciences' Institute of Medicine was in the midst of revis-
ing all RDAs to reflect current thinking, distinguishing

the needs of different age groups. On this latter score I should note some clinicians have been thinking for a long time that vitamin A's RDA is too *high* for older people. (See, e.g., R.M. Russell, "Vitamin Requirements of Elderly People; an Update," *American Journal of Clinical Nutrition* 1993; 58:4–14).

Incidentally, the therapeutic effects of vitamin A, as well as practically all the antioxidant nutrients discussed in this chapter, are said to be greater when used with one another.

2. B Complex

Most of the vitamins in the B complex are considered to assist in the treatment of peripheral neuropathy, especially when taken in combination.

(a) B1 (thiamin)

Some medical professionals believe that **B1** or **thiamin** is particularly useful in **improving nerve function** and **diminishing pain**. The Atkins Institute for Complementary Medicine reports a 50% benefit rate for their patients suffering from diabetic neuropathy when thiamin is given in injections. The Institute also refers to a supporting 12-week German study where B1 (together with other B vitamins) was given in high dosages—320 mg daily—to patients with diabetic neuropathy (V. Frydl et al., *Medwelt*, 1989; 40: 1484–86). Other doctors have reportedly found that a high percentage of their PN diabetic patients have achieved improvements with daily thiamin dosages in the 50–100 mg range. (A few suggest, however, there may be no measurable benefit in treating neurological disorders with thiamin unless there was a thiamin deficiency to begin with, as may often be caused by excessive alcohol intake.[2])

Recommended dosages vary widely. The RDA for thiamin is 1.2 to 1.5 milligrams for males, 1.0 to 5 for women. Some therapeutic recommendations, though, go as high as 50 to 100 milligrams daily and occasionally even more (see above).

(b) B2 (riboflavin)

This vitamin is important in the production of **body energy**. The special significance of **B2** to us, though, lies in its ability to both help with the conversion of B6 to a form we can use and help generate **glutathione**. The latter is an enzyme which acts as one of our most significant antioxidants. (This enzyme is a carefully designed molecule of protein which can "quench" free radicals but needs vitamin E, the mineral selenium, and other factors in order to do its work.)

A deficiency of riboflavin can result in **nerve disorders** and a **degeneration of myelin sheaths**. It works closely with folic acid, pantothenic acid (vitamin B5) and vitamin B12. It can also lessen the symptoms of pantothenic acid and zinc deficiencies.

---

[2] One neurologist told me that a steady diet of polished rice, which is thiamin deficient, can result in neuropathy.

The RDA for riboflavin is 1.7 mg daily for adults. Those who exercise are said to require 2 to 2.5 mg daily. Users of medications such as Elavil and Tofranil, discussed previously, are sometimes counseled to take up to 10 mg each day.

(c) B3 (niacin)

Niacin is often used to reduce **high cholesterol** levels and treat high blood pressure, acne and alcoholism. It is also recommended for **weight reduction** since it helps stabilize blood sugar levels. The particular importance to us is its reported assistance in **improving circulation** and in the **proper functioning of the nervous system**. Dr. Lark Lands, in her book, *Positively Well: Living With HIV as a Chronic, Manageable Survival Disease* (now out-of-print), mentions niacin favorably as one of the B complex members particularly helpful in **rebuilding the myelin sheath** around nerves of HIV patients afflicted with PN.

A review panel under the auspices of the National Academy of Sciences' Institute of Medicine recently indicated that niacin could be used at doses up to 35 mg a day before side effects such as flushing were incurred. However, some practitioners have prescribed the vitamin at levels as high as one to three grams a day for therapeutic purposes. Anyone considering levels higher than 35 mg daily, particularly people with diabetes (because of possible effects on blood sugar levels), should consult their doctor first.

(d) B5 (pantothenic acid)

This is considered one of the best **energy enhancing** vitamins and is also valued for its **anti-inflammatory** properties. In a 1997 study at the Munchener Medizin-ische Wochenschrift in Germany, reported by the Life Extension Foundation, 28 out of 33 patients who had been treated solely with alpha-lipoic acid (more on that nutrient later) for PN showed further improvement when vitamin **B5** was added to the treatment.

For general health it's been suggested that 100 to 200 milligrams per day might be appropriate. Increases beyond that to the 600 to 1200 mg range, which is a therapeutic dosage, should be under a doctor's supervision.

(e) B6 (pyridoxine)

B6 is important in manufacturing **prostaglandins**, hormonal compounds that assist in the transport of oxygen in the blood stream. Pyridoxine is also considered to influence the nervous system through its effects on neurotransmitters. High dosages, however can be toxic and can actually **cause** peripheral neuropathy. The RDA is two milligrams for adults. Some doctors think up to 50 milligrams may be taken daily without concern and that a definite PN occurring risk doesn't usually occur until daily dosages exceed 200 milligrams. On the other hand, at least a few neurologists would limit the daily intake of B6 to 25 mg for people with PN currently.

In spite of cautions concerning excessive usage of B6, at least one clinical study indicates clear benefits when the vitamin is taken in adequate amounts, particularly when it's used in combination with B1. In a 1997 investigation conducted at the Muhimbili University College of Health Sciences in Tanzania and reported in the *East African Medical Journal* (1997 Dec. 74 [12]: 803–8), the clinical response to therapeutic doses of the two vitamins taken together were determined in 200 diabetic patients with "symptomatic" peripheral neuropathy. One hundred were randomly allocated to group A and given B1 at 25 mg/day and B6 at 50 mg/day. The rest were assigned to group B where they were given an identical appearing tablet daily but which contained only one mg each of the two vitamins. Four weeks after starting treatment the severity of signs of peripheral neuropathy reportedly decreased in 48.9% of patients in group A compared with 11.4% in group B, indicating a much higher benefit rate when therapeutic dosages are used.

(f) B12 (cobalamin)

In addition to contributing to the **metabolism of nerve tissue**, vitamin **B12** helps guard against stroke and heart disease and is said to contribute to relief from asthma, depression and low blood pressure.

B12 is thought to be one of the most effective members of the B complex for us PNers. Dr. Sheldon Hendler, a noted expert in vitamin therapies, reports that in a series of 39 patients treated for neurologic symptoms related to B12 deficiency, all showed improvement from taking the nutrient. Other studies have demonstrated that aggressive B12 therapy eases pain from the nerve damage of diabetic neuropathy. The flip side of this is that deficiencies of the vitamin can directly lead to peripheral neuropathy. (An article in a 1996 issue of *Nutrition Reviews* reported that "vitamin B12 deficiency is linked to peripheral neuropathy in 40% of cases.") One of the more common tests for PN, in fact, is to determine the level of cobalamin in a patient's blood.

Vitamin B12 is considered quite safe in even large amounts. Daily maintenance dosage for general health is put by some authorities at 100 to 200 micrograms (mcg) daily although the RDA is 6 mcg. For deficiency problems it's sometimes suggested that at least one mg (1000 mcg) be taken daily.

Vitamin B12 is frequently given by **muscle injections** since this enhances absorption by the body. In fact some practitioners suggest that with any condition requiring speedy and direct relief such as neuropathy, intramuscular injections on a weekly or monthly basis are the preferred method of administration over pills.

(g) Biotin

Biotin is essential for **cell growth** and replication through its role in the manufacture of the nucleic acids DNA and RNA, which make up the genetic material of the cell.

It is ordinarily taken in doses from 30 to 300 mcg daily. There is some evidence, however, that megadosages can be effective in improving nerve conduction and relieving PN pain. In a study performed at the University of Athens, subjects with PN were given 10 mg by intramuscular injection three times a week for six weeks, followed by 5 mg daily taken orally. Within four to eight weeks symptoms were reported to have decreased significantly (specifically painful muscle cramps, *paresthesias*, ability to stand, walk and climb stairs, and disappearance of restless leg syndrome in all patients) with no adverse side effects. Dr. Lark Lands, who reported the study, suggests that taking 10–15 mg of biotin daily, in conjunction with other B vitamins, might prove useful in improving nerve function.

Biotin is said to work closely with folic acid, pantothenic acid and vitamin B12 and lessen the symptoms of pantothenic acid and zinc deficiencies.

(h) Folic Acid

Also referred to as **folate**, **folic acid** is said to rank number one in vitamin deficiency in North America. It is involved in a large number of **metabolic processes**, perhaps the most important being the **synthesis of DNA**. Folic acid is considered helpful in the maintenance of nerve cells.

The RDA for folic acid is 400 mcg daily and it is often used in conjunction with vitamin B12. Similarly to that vitamin and biotin, folate is occasionally given intramuscularly by injection for PN. In these instances it reportedly has been administered in dosages as high as 20–60 mg, or 50 or more times the RDA specification.

(i) Inositol

This nutrient, found naturally in the body, perhaps should be regarded as a distant relative rather than a direct family member of the B complex. Some people take the nutritionally active form called **myoinositol** as a supplement in one or two gram amounts daily to help them sleep better or to reduce their nervous tension.

Decreased levels of **inositol** are found in nerve cells of people with diabetes. This reduced level may be partially responsible for diabetic PN. Apparently a high degree of blood glucose causes a build up of a chemical known as **sorbitol** in nerve cells while at the same time decreasing the inositol.

In one reported investigation involving 20 diabetic patients with peripheral neuropathy, 1650 milligrams of myoinositol were given daily with researchers noting improved sensory nerve function. In another study researchers at the University of Alabama found a statistically significant improvement in nerve function among diabetic patients placed on a diet high in inositol, including such high-inositol foods as cantaloupe, peanuts, grapefruit and whole grains. Dr. Robert Atkins has reported success in treating peripheral neuropathy with two to six grams of myoinositol daily; he notes that physicians at St. James Hospital in Leeds, England, have reported good results with smaller dosages.

In spite of these reports, people with diabetes are advised to be under a doctor's supervision when considering the supplemental use of myoinositol.

(j) Choline and Lecithin

Lecithin as sold in health stores contains **phosphatidylcholine** (generally referred to simply as **PC**) which is a protector of cells in our nervous systems. PC itself is a source of **choline** which in turn forms yet another chemical in our bodies called **acetylcholine**. This latter chemical is an important neurotransmitter which is said to mediate emotions and behavior.

Although I found no direct reference to the use of PC or choline for PN, there are indications these chemicals contribute to the production of myelin, the covering which protects nerves. There is also ample evidence that these nutrients can be helpful in treating various neurological disorders such as Parkinson's disease and Tourette syndrome.

Practitioners suggest that in most cases up to 10 grams per day of PC or one gram per day of choline can be safely taken to good effect. Doses higher than these should probably be taken only under a doctor's supervision.

(k) B Combinations

Before leaving the subject of B vitamins it should again be stressed that they should be taken as a group to assure their **synergistic action** and to prevent imbalance. In one study seeming to support this idea clinically (performed at St. Marienhospital, Lunen, Germany, and reported in the October 20, 1992, issue of *Fortschrifte der Medizin*), various therapeutic combinations of vitamins

B2, B6 and B12 were considered. It was an investigation reportedly involving 234 doctors in private practices treating 1149 patients with polyneuropathy, neuralgia, radiculopathy (a pathological condition of the nerve roots), neuritis associated with pain and *paresthesias* (sensations). The end points evaluated were intensity of pain, muscle weakness affecting legs, and *paresthesia*. The study concluded there was a clear improvement in these symptoms from the use of these combinations. At a second examination approximately three weeks after initiation of treatments, a positive effect on pain in particular was said to have been observed in 69% of the cases. Similar observations were also made for *paresthesias* and muscular weakness in the legs.

Dr. Ward Dean, author of the book, *Smart Drugs and Nutrients,* mentions a 1996 double-blind study of 24 diabetic patients who suffered from PN in which a high-dose B complex regimen was used: thiamin, 320 mg/day for the first 2 weeks, and 120 mg/d thereafter; vitamin B6, 720 mg/d for the first 2 weeks, and 270 mg/d thereafter; and vitamin B12 2000 mcg/d for the first 2 weeks and then 750 mcg/d thereafter. According to the principal investigator, the treatment resulted in significant improvement in nerve conduction velocity in the peroneal nerve (a small nerve associated with the fibula and innervating certain muscle and skin areas of the leg and foot) and an improvement of the "vibration perception threshold."

You can find combinations of the Bs in various strengths at any health food store packaged as "B complex" vitamins. Be *sure*, though, that folate and adequate levels of B12 are included in the formulation. Otherwise you may wish to consider adding them separately— as I do.

3. Vitamin C (ascorbic acid)

Scurvy, the vitamin **C** deficiency disease, has been recognized for at least a couple of thousand years but it was not until the 16th century that people realized certain fruits and vegetables could prevent or cure it. In the late 18th century English sailors carried limes on long voyages to ward off scurvy which led to them being nicknamed "limeys."

Vitamin C or **ascorbic acid** is one of the most powerful antioxidants known. In addition to the direct benefit it provides in fighting free radicals, vitamin C specifically complements the action of other nutrients such as PC and choline just discussed, as well as vitamin E, glutathione and selenium. In fact high levels of vitamin C appear to increase blood levels of most antioxidants. Vitamin C also plays a role in the manufacture of neurotransmitters.

Studies performed at the University of Scranton and reported in *High-Speed Healing* (authored by the editors of *Prevention Magazine*) found that vitamin C can also reduce the concentration of sorbitol, a type of sugar, in red blood cells as mentioned earlier and in this way protect against diabetic neuropathy.

Adequate levels of ascorbic acid are considered indispensable for good health. A National Health and

Nutrition Examination Survey looked at the vitamin C intake of over 11,000 people during a five-year period. Results showed that those in the high vitamin C intake group (greater than 50 mg daily) had a *48%* lower chance of death from all causes than those in the low intake group (less than 50 mg daily).

The RDA for this vitamin was set long ago at 60 mg but it is now generally felt that most people could do well to supplement their regular diets with at least 500 to 1000 mg (1 gram) per day. Some practitioners in fact suggest dosages as high as five to ten grams daily to treat particular disorders or to boost the body's immune system.

4. Vitamin E

Vitamin **E** is said to be the oldest biologic antioxidant and is considered particularly important for **heart health**. In one investigation, dubbed CHAOS for Cambridge Heart Antioxidant Study, 2002 men and women with artery narrowings who were participating were given either 400 or 800 IUs of vitamin E or a placebo daily. A statistical analysis following the study showed that vitamin E cut the risk of heart attack by more than half and the risk of a nonfatal heart attack by 77%.

Vitamin E **protects cell membranes** and plays a crucial role in **immune defenses**. The importance of this vitamin to us is that it also **sustains normal neurological processes**, particularly in its **alpha-tocopherol** form. A 1997 study reported in the *American Family Physician* suggested that a serious deficiency of vitamin E can have a profound effect on the central nervous system, leading to significant muscle weakness and visual field constriction.

Another study performed at the Institute of Chemical Pathology at Tel Hashomer in Israel in 1995 indicated that children with vitamin E deficiencies who had neuropathies and who were treated with intramuscular and oral administrations of vitamin E were significantly benefited.

The RDA for vitamin E is 30 IUs. Many practitioners, however, recommend anywhere from 400 to 800 IUs per day. In a recent issue of the *Harvard Heart Letter*, some members of the editorial board, certainly a conservative group, say "the case for taking vitamin E in a dosage of 200 to 800 IUs per day is reasonable, and getting stronger."

Vitamin E exerts enhanced antioxidant effects in combination with other antioxidants including beta carotene, vitamin C and selenium. It also regulates levels of vitamin A and in fact is necessary for the action of vitamin A. In addition it may be required for the conversion of vitamin B12 to its active form and may reduce some of the symptoms of zinc deficiency.

[comments re vitamins are not to be considered medical opinions and should not be relied upon as such—always consult your doctor:

(1) Peripheral neuropathy is sometimes caused by a lack of **vitamins B**. Maybe your husband did not care about his intake of vitamin B for years. Alcohol or some pills (e.g. Tegretol) may be responsible for a vitamin B neuropathy. Even if vitamin B levels are normal in a blood test, this

does not mean that a severe lack of vitamin B could not have caused the neuropathy long before, and the nervous system seems to need enormous amounts of vitamin B to recover from the damage (re myelinization, that is filling up the gaps in the sheaths of the nerves). I successfully treated somebody with a disabling neuropathy with injections (every 2 weeks) of a mixture of vitamins B1, B6 and B12 (Neurorubin Streuli, Swiss trade mark) for a year, and symptoms disappeared almost completely apart from a feeling of stiff ankles in the morning. Naturally one could take vitamin pills, but sometimes even the intestinal absorption of vitamins is disturbed by the lack of vitamin B, and then one has to start with injections, but TAKE CARE TO AVOID HYPERVITAMINOSIS (pause the treatment from time to time). If the neuropathy of your husband is accompanied by pain, injections of vitamin B can make them disappear immediately (2–3 injections/week). This is a very common problem, but most doctors rely too much on lab-values of vitamin B and hesitate to start a vitamin therapy even if the symptoms are typical. Karin

(2) I have painful feet and take half a tablet of **niacin** every night and sleep well with it . . . don't know why it works but it does! Bruce

(3) I have written before about **B6** and PN. According to the drs at Penn Univ in Phila, the medical journals contain articles with evidence of B6 induced PN. I have another medical condition and my hematologist wanted to treat me with 100 milligrams of B6 twice a day and **folic acid**. My neurologist at Penn was adamantly against anymore than 25 milligrams of B6 per day for a PN patient. He said folic acid was fine in a high dose but NOT B6. The drs. at Penn are actively involved in PN research which is currently funded by the Muscular Dystrophy Assoc. My dr. in particular researches the gene-based PN which runs in families

and has no particular cause. He said they have isolated about 7 genes and are constantly working in the research of PN. Vitamin therapy is risky without consulting a neurologist that is highly involved in PN treatment. My hematologist had no idea B6 could cause or aggravate PN. After talking with my Penn dr. he was convinced of the potential complications resulting from B6. Whether other medical professionals agree with the drs. at Penn is unknown to me. I have a great deal of respect for Penn Univ drs. and the research they are doing. Anon

(4) It looks like doctors all over the country have different opinions. My neurologist suggested I take only 50mg [of **B6**], but that was after he had my regular doctor run some blood tests. I also read or heard on TV that too much B-6 was not good for you but no recommendation was made as to what was the correct dosage. I'll play it safe, I hope, and go along with my doctor. Marilyn

(5) I have taken 250 Mcg caps of **B-12** for over a year now. While I still have deep leg pain the burning in my feet has subsided at least 75%. Woody

(6) I am taking 1000 mg. of Vitamin **B 12** for about 6 months. Helps the pain a little. Anon

(7) I never took a vitamin in my life until the last couple of years. I started off with **Vitamin B100** [assume a complex is meant] simply because the doc said that lack of vitamin B can contribute to PN. After my two years on heavy doses of antidepressant and various pain meds, I switched my treatment plan to include vitamins and minerals. To tell you the truth, I don't know if the vitamins are helping or not. I have no way to determine what the "normal" progression of this crazy disease is. Questions as to whether it would have progressed faster or slower, if I would be in more or less pain . . . who knows. I do know that my general

health has improved. Was it the vitamins or the fact that I'm no longer working and living a stress-free (well, somewhat) life . . . again who knows. My doctor keeps telling me there was no reason for my PN other than a mutant gene. I go in with a list each time . . . could it have been exposure to some chemical, could it have been X-rays, could it have been drug reaction of some kind . . . I go CRAZY with trying figure out the why and how. I wish it could be something easy like vitamins, or lack of vitamins. It would be a great comfort to me to be able to pin this disease on something. Why did this happen? What caused my body to start destroying the peripheral nerves? Why did it progress so fast? I have a vision . . . someday a doctor will pour purple liquid into a beaker and orange smoke will curl upward . . . he will shout "Eureka . . . I've found the answer to Peripheral Neuropathy." Doctors will gather around and shake their heads and say "Damn, is THAT all it was? Why didn't we think of THAT." Someday. Dotti

(8) I am 42 yrs old with polyneuropathy. All blood work came back fine. I started taking vitamins, even though no deficiency showed up in my blood. The vitamins are **E**, **super B-50**, **1000 mg C**, and iron. The B has 500mg **folic acid** in it. Also I started the Chroma slim 1,2,3 to help take off some weight. Well, the chroma #3 has 400 mg folic acid, which I take 3 times a day. Add it all up and I am taking 1400 mg folic acid a day. Third week into it, my energy is way up!!!!! I now have some pain free days!!!!! Had my emg done yesterday, some of my nerves went from a slow speed of 30 last emg to a speed of 50 this time; the norm for my age is 60!!!!!! So hey you guys out there ask your doctors about it. I hope I do not speak too soon. Joyce

(9) When I started getting serious foot pain from Diabetic PN, I found a message in a diabetic forum recommending taking **Choline** (1200 mg daily) and **Lecithin** (2500 mg).

I've been doing so for about 3 years now. It seems to help. Best indication is on dàys when I forget to take them, the pain is worse. I also rub on Capsaicin cream (available OTC in various brands now) 3–4 times a day. If I forget that before I go to bed, nighttime pain is worse, so it also seems to work. Bruce

(10) I take **Vitamin E** in 400 IU doses. I usually take 2 or 3 in the morning and the same amount at night. I really notice when I have been off Vitamin E, the PN and pain in my legs, feet and arms gets much worse. It usually take 2 weeks before I start noticing any changes. Once I started taking Vitamin E again it really did help. Thanks Bill!]

Minerals

Minerals are labeled inorganic nutrients because they contain no carbon. Of the 60 found in the body, only about 22 are considered essential to human nutrition. These help preserve heart, brain, muscle and nerve systems.

Similarly to vitamins, many minerals function as coenzymes, acting as catalysts for biologic reactions such as muscle response, digestion and the transmission of messages through the nervous system.

The particular minerals which are most important to PNers are thought to be selenium, magnesium, chromium and zinc.

1. Selenium

Selenium is a powerful **antioxidant**. Additionally, it serves as a constituent of the enzyme **glutathione**

peroxidase, which interacts with vitamin E in preventing free radicals from stealing electrons away from healthy cells. Selenium also reinforces the body's immune defenses. (People infected with the HIV virus frequently suffer from a selenium deficiency.) Moreover, it has **anti-inflammatory** properties, reinforced when taken in conjunction with vitamin E and other vitamin antioxidants.

Selenium is considered a "**trace**" mineral because it's needed only in minute amounts—micrograms rather than milligrams. Some practitioners suggest a daily intake of 200–400 mcg for therapeutic purposes. However, for simple general health maintenance, the editors of the *UC Berkeley Wellness Letter* in their April 1997 issue contended that most people get as much selenium as they need from their regular diets and that a multi-vitamin/mineral pill containing selenium taken daily should be sufficient in any event.

2. Magnesium

Magnesium is known to be necessary for **nerve conduction** as well as for protein synthesis and for the anaerobic breakdown of glucose. The mineral is also vital for thiamin, vitamin C and pyridoxine metabolism.

A few practitioners have found that magnesium deficiencies either cause peripheral neuropathy or are associated with PN. For example, in a study of 128 patients with Type 2 diabetes conducted at the Department of Medicine, Bahia Federal University Medical School,

Brazil, and reported in a May 1998 issue of *Diabetes Care*, magnesium levels were found to be significantly lower in patients with peripheral neuropathy than in those in a control group.

Dr. Sally Stroud of the Houston Immunological Institute in Texas has found magnesium supplements help correct some neuropathies. In patients with decreased serum magnesium levels, she reports intravenous supplementation followed by oral augmentation decreased neuropathic sensations and the use of pain medications.

Some doctors suggest adding 200 to 400 milligrams of supplemental magnesium daily to one's diet. Dr. Mildred Seelig, a well-known magnesium researcher, would go further and reportedly has recommended a daily intake of 6 to 10 mg per kg of body weight per day for optimal health.

3. Chromium

Chromium is essential for normal **sugar metabolism**. It works with insulin to move glucose into cells where it can be used to generate energy. Optimal chromium intake appears to decrease the amount of insulin needed to maintain normal blood sugar. Chromium also acts with insulin to stimulate **protein synthesis**.

Like selenium, chromium is regarded as a trace mineral, requiring only small supplemental amounts. Although its role with PN is less well defined than that of selenium or magnesium, there are doctors who suspect its deficiency in the body may also contribute to peripheral neuropathy. These practitioners recommend 200 to 400 *micrograms* of chromium daily be added to a neuropathy therapy program. (Doctors at the Department of Medicine, St. Michael's Hospital, in Ontario, Canada, in 1996 found that the infusion of 250 micrograms of trivalent chromium daily into a patient who had peripheral neuropathy of the axonal type and was glucose intolerant resulted in the "remission" of the neuropathy four days after the infusions were begun!)

4. Zinc

Zinc functions in over 200 **enzymatic reactions** in the body and is involved in the synthesis and conversion of carbohydrates, lipids and proteins to useable forms. It is also necessary for the production of brain neurotransmitters.

Deficiency of zinc in the body is said to lead to impaired conduction and nerve damage. Dr. Robert Atkins of the Atkins Center for Complementary Medicine claims that zinc deficiency is implicated in a whole range of neurological and neuropsychiatric disorders. Although no specific studies were found involving human subjects, a 1993 investigation at the Department of Biochemistry, University of Missouri, indicated zinc deficiency in chicks and guinea pigs correlated with signs of peripheral neuropathy and that they were readily reversed by zinc therapy.

Dr. Atkins indicates that a daily therapeutic dose of 15–25 mg of zinc should be sufficient for most people. Incidentally, zinc is considered toxic in large doses and can cause nausea and diarrhea. It also has been suggested that if any zinc supplementation is carried on over a long period of time copper supplementation should be undertaken as well since copper could be depleted in the body. Experts say that many multi-vitamin pills probably contain sufficient copper for this purpose.

[comments re minerals are not to be considered medical opinions and should not be relied upon as such—always consult your doctor:

(1) I, too, got peripheral neuropathy from d4t. After a stint on sustained release morphine, I switched to **magnesium** supplements and lipoic acid supplementation and got noticeable relief (i.e. full function with minor tingling). M

(2) I was diagnosed in October with PN (through EMG and nerve conduction tests) after typical symptoms—numb hands and feet, imbalance, etc. Blood work all fine, so cause at this point is not known. One theory the neurologist had was the high amount of **selenium** in the multi-vitamin I was taking. There subsequently was an article in TIME magazine titled "Vitamin Overload?" (Nov. 10, 1997). I've stopped taking the vitamins, and am waiting to go back for another EMG, etc. in January to see if there is any change, but so far things have not gotten better, and now there is pain and burning in addition to the numbness. Anne

(3) I too, have terrible back pain when I stand in one spot for more than 3 min. I get leg cramps when my magnesium gets low. I then take a **calcium**, **magnesium** and **zinc** tablet—you have to take the combination for it to work properly. After several days, my legs are o.k. Wish I could find as easy a solution for my back! My doctor just says, "I

know, I know" and gives me another prescription for pain meds.! Nancy]

Herbs

Frowned on by the medical community for a long time, the plants and plant components known as **herbs** are now being accepted by many (but certainly not all) doctors as useful therapeutical adjuncts. This growing acceptance seems inevitable considering that about a quarter of today's conventional medications were derived from herbs: for example aspirin from white willow bark and digitalis drugs from foxglove. And even though science is frequently not able to pin down and calibrate the effects of herbal compounds there seems to be plenty of anecdotal evidence showing usage benefits.

The public certainly seems to have embraced herbs. In fact more than one-third of all Americans are said to presently use herbal medicine for some aspect of primary health care.

It should be cautioned that many herbs contain a variety of active ingredients which can have profound effects—for better or worse—on people. One point made is that some of these over-the-counter "**phytomedicines**" could have troublesome interactions with other drugs and should only be taken under a doctor's supervision. Nevertheless reported adverse reactions are rare.

Incidentally, the Dietary Supplement Health and Education Act (DSHEA) of 1994 permits herbs to be sold legally so long as no claims for **disease treatment** are made on the product label. The FDA in fact has adopted regulations keeping *any* health claims off the label unless there is **"significant scientific agreement"** that the claims are valid. (The Supreme Court recently upheld these regulations in a challenge to their constitutionality.) It should be noted that under DSHEA there is no legal requirement of **product standardization** for herbs or for their **safety** or **efficacy**.

Some medical practitioners urge that herbs be fully regulated. For example in a June 1998 editorial in the prestigious *New England Journal of Medicine*, the argument is made that herbal remedies should be subjected to the same rigorous standards as mainstream treatments.[3] The authors contend: "There cannot be two kinds of medicine—conventional and alternative."

A fair question, it seems to me, is why not?—as long as the consumer understands that herbs have not been reviewed for safety and efficacy. In making a judgment on whether these remedies should be subjected to the same standards as conventional medications (sometimes referred to as allopathic medicine), one needs to weigh the cost of putting them through the FDA's extraordinarily lengthy and expensive review process (estimated as high as $200 million per approved drug) against the limited

---

[3] The application of mainstream standards is certainly no guaranty that an approved drug is any safer than an unapproved herb. Late in 1998, for example, the new diabetes drug Rezulin, which had recently received the go-ahead from the FDA, was found linked to 33 deaths.

benefits the review process would provide. This is particularly true when you consider that practically all herbal
remedies have experienced a long history of safe and (at
least anecdotally reported) effective use.

The review process would add a cost factor to herbs
that undoubtedly would prove unacceptable to consumers. Surely since nutrient manufacturers have no or
little patent protection it would be unimaginable that
many, or any, would make the required investments to
find out whether, in the end, the customer would pay the
necessarily sharply higher price. It should be kept in
mind that the customer could go to many other places in
the world and buy the same product at the old price.

Usually when medical practitioners argue for more
regulation they point to the hype often associated with
nutrient marketing. Certainly there have been abuses in
this regard. However, effectively eliminating herbal
remedies from the marketplace by imposing an expensive review process and depriving users of their benefits
is too extreme an answer to excessive sales pitches in my
opinion. In any event new guidelines adopted late in
1998 by the Federal Trade Commission should take care
of any problems in this regard—guidelines which appear
to reinforce the DSHEA standards mentioned earlier.
Manufacturers of dietary supplements must now provide
scientific evidence to substantiate claims if they are
made based on **traditional uses**. Further, they are to be
held accountable for the **"net impression"** of their ad-
vertising and will be held responsible for substantiating
each reasonable interpretation. One example given is

that if a manufacturer runs an ad claiming 90% of cardiologists regularly take a product, it must be able to support its implied claim that the product offers some benefit to the heart.

With that out of the way, following are some of the herbs and herbal derivatives that have been used for dealing with peripheral neuropathy.

1. Ginkgo Biloba

Ginkgo biloba is an extract made from leaves of the tree bearing the same name. The tree, also called the maidenhair tree, is said to belong to a species at least 300 million years old.

Ginkgo biloba's principal therapeutic value arises from its **antioxidant properties**. There is also evidence that it helps in cases of impaired mental performance and enhances short-term memory by regulating **neurotransmission**. In fact the extract has been shown to be effective in both the prevention and early intervention of CNS disorders associated with aging. In this respect it appears to act by facilitating better blood flow through the body and especially through the brain.

In Europe ginkgo biloba has become one of the most frequently prescribed medications. Reportedly, there have been more than 50 double-blind clinical studies performed there showing its favorable effects on both vascular insufficiency and age-related decreases in brain function.

A 1993 study examined the efficacy of a component of ginkgo biloba in small mammals. In an experimental model designed to mimic peripheral neuropathy based on traumatic damage to sciatic nerves, results showed improved functional nerve regeneration.

An analysis of 15 European studies on the herb was reported in the November–December 1998 issue of *Archives of Family Medicine* in an article, "A Review of 12 Commonly Used Medicinal Herbs." The report indicated ginkgo biloba caused an overall reduction in claudication (lameness or limping) symptoms of the subjects examined and permitted a 50% increase in their pain-free walking. (Although many PNers certainly can relate to the walking part, it wasn't clear from the article whether the problems experienced by the subjects had been circulatory or neurological.)

Some practitioners suggest taking 120–160 mg daily of this herb for general mental acuity and up to 240–360 mg daily for therapeutic purposes. Nevertheless, the authors of the *Family Medicine* article suggest limiting the intake to 120 mg per day of standardized ginkgo (designated Egb 761).

Ginkgo is generally considered quite safe. However, it has been linked to stroke in a very few cases, demonstrating again the desirability of consulting with your doctor before taking herbal remedies such as this.

2. St. John's Wort

St. John's wort (SJW) is a plant which grows in the wild (at one time it inhabited over two million acres in northern California) and is harvested for its active ingredient, **hypericum**. Its principal use is as a natural herbal alternative to **antidepressant** medications such as Prozac, Paxil and Zoloft.

The efficacy of hypericum as a treatment for mild or moderate depression has been validated by a number of European studies, including those performed at the Centre for Complementary Health Studies at Exeter in the U.K., at Sodra in Stockholm, Sweden, and at Ludwig-Maximilians University in Munich, Germany. (In Germany, in fact, it has been reported to out-sell the leading antidepressant, Prozac, 20 to 1.)[4] In many studies hypericum side effects were found to be less troublesome than with traditional antidepressants, the principal one being an increased **photosensitization** or sensitivity to sunlight. But even this problem is not particularly common, generally being limited to fair skinned individuals taking large dosages.

There have been few reported investigations concerning the use of SJW for PN patients although it is frequently suggested as a treatment. An August 1988 issue of *AIDS Treatment News* reported interviews of 11 AIDs victims with peripheral neuropathy who had taken hypericum for approximately three months. Nine reported beneficial results.

The federal Office of Complementary and Alternative Medicine has allocated $4.3 million to determine long-

---

[4] The Germans are world leaders in dealing with the medicinal aspects of herbs. For the past three decades the German Health Authority has systematically reviewed evidence on about 300 herbs and formulated clinical guidelines for their use.

term side effects of SJW as well as optimal dosage and relative safety and efficacy. The study began in 1998 and is to continue for three years.

Although the mechanism of action is not completely understood, there is some speculation that, in dealing with PN, St. John's wort may act like tricyclic antidepressants such as Elavil and Tofranil discussed earlier.

There are strict warnings that this herb should not be used with other antidepressants because of **toxicity** factors. The daily dosage, when it may be taken, is suggested by some practitioners as two to four grams of the powdered herb or two tenths to one gram of the powdered extract. The authors of the *Family Medicine* article cited above suggest 300 mg three times a day of an SJW extract standardized to 0.3% hypericum.

3. Bioflavonoids

Bioflavonoids are pigment substances found in many plants where they impart color to flowers, leaves and stems. They are considered excellent **antioxidants** both individually and in combination with vitamin C.

A Hungarian researcher who won the Nobel Prize in Medicine (for among other things his discovery of vitamin C) named these substances vitamin P many years ago—a name which didn't last for long. Interestingly, another researcher born in Hungary more recently has espoused bioflavonoids for the treatment of **diabetic nerve** conditions. Dr. Zoltan P. Rona, author of *The Joy of Health* and the medical editor of the *Encyclopedia of*

Natural Healing claims that bioflavonoids such as quercetin, pycnogenol, hesperidin, catechin, and rutin safely and effectively inhibit the enzyme aldose reductase. This inhibition can be important in the treatment of diabetic peripheral neuropathy (more about this later).

Bioflavonoids are often supplemented as a group in amounts of 250 to 500 mg, one to several times daily. Many vitamin C formulas contain bioflavonoids, particularly rutin and hesperidin. Quercetin is available in various strengths; supplementation of 100 to 250 mg three times daily is considered an effective level by some proponents.

4. Other Herbs and Herbal Derivatives

There are a number of other herbal compounds which have been suggested for treating peripheral neuropathy in addition to those discussed here (as well as cayenne and mugwort, previously mentioned).

Grape seed extract is one of the more prominent. It's sold in most health food stores and is said by its proponents to be 20 times more powerful than vitamin C and 50 times stronger than vitamin E as an antioxidant. Some researchers attribute the surprising fact that the French enjoy half the heart disease rate of Americans, in spite of their penchant for rich sauces and fatty products known to contribute to heart disease, to the fact they drink so much more grape wine than we do.

The herb **goshajinkigan** is said to have been long used in Japan to alleviate diabetic neuropathy. In a study at the University of Yamanashi Medical School in

1994 involving 13 patients with diabetic neuropathy, the researchers concluded that the administration of 7.5 grams daily of goshajinkigan for three months relieved subjective symptoms and improved sensations in 9 of the 13. (Reported in *Diabetes Research and Clinical Practice*, December 16, 1994.)

Other herbal remedies frequently mentioned for PN include **cat's claw** (said to have powerful antioxidant and anti-inflammatory properties); **feverfew** (claimed to block or reduce inflammatory reactions); **ginseng** (considered to be a mild sedative and tonic to nerve centers); **green tea** (like grape seed extract said to be an even more powerful antioxidant than vitamins C or E); **hops flower** (said to have a relaxing effect upon the central nervous system); **Noni plant** fruit or juice (a tropical plant known in the Caribbean as the "pain killer tree" and valued for its analgesic properties); and **valerian root** (used for depression and thought to help with anxiety, nervous sleeplessness and muscle cramping, as well as pain relief).

On a lighter note I came across the following substance being sold for diabetic neuropathy. In addition to St. John's wort and ginkgo biloba this product has several ingredients which sound miraculous including phosphorous for relief from "burning" (I always thought phosphorous made things burn!), plumbum for "shooting neuralgic pains," carbovegetabilis for "the need to be fanned or sticking feet out from under the bed covers," agaricus for "shivering" (maybe sticking those tootsies out from a warm bed gives you the shivers), and allium for "traumatic neuralgia." You get one ounce of all of this plus nine other herbal ingredients which are said to help with everything from menopause disorders to varicose veins, for only $14! (And you don't even have to go to the carnival to buy it.)

[comments re herbs are not to be considered medical opinions and should not be relied upon as such— always consult your doctor:

(1) I have been taking Gengko (**Ginkgo Biloba**) for about six weeks. I started it because it was supposed to improve one's memory. It hasn't done a darn thing for me, including relieving any PN pain! Jenny

(2) I just underwent a lumbar laminectomy in September, and after suffering a great deal of pain from neuropathy by an EMG prior to surgery, I have found significant relief from taking 50 mg. Nortriptyline 2x daily, along with tonic water, and something called Isotonix OPC-3 by Health Power, distributed by Market America, Inc, Greensboro, NC 27409, a powder derivative from extracts from **grape seeds, red wine, pine bark, bilberry and citrus.** I am usually most skeptical about such products, but am living proof that such a product has helped both of us, and may secure significant results for you. Michael

(3) Well, I am having excellent results with a Neurontin/ zoloft/**St John's Wort** combination. Hands are in remission, and feet are itching/burning infrequently now. So far knock on wood, I am living a pretty pain-free life since trying this combination. BTW it is 4800mg Neurontin, 50mg zoloft and 1000mg St John's Wort. Yes that's 4800mg Neurontin—12 pills a day,and I would double it again if it helped. I do have a doctor who I can tell that I am not satisfied with results and let's try something else. Thank God for that. Di

(4) I am not taking any other [than **St. John's wort**] anti-depressant drugs. I have been taking 1 300 MG pill a day and yesterday I felt great. Pain level down a lot. So far so good. Anon

(5) I now take **St. John's Wort** and **hops**; in addition, a posting on this BB recommended 400 IU of Vitamin E 3 times a day. This combination is helping me. I've tried eliminating one or the other and feel a difference. Some people have posted good results with cayenne pepper (capsule form) and its counterpart in a topical cream Capsaicin. I found the former ineffective, the latter pure torture. You've just got to keep trying things until you find some that take the edge off. Marjorie

(6) I take 100mg of Ultram 4xday /and 800 mg neurontin 4xday . . . but something else also helped me a great deal and that was **grape seed extract** . . . it is an antioxidant. I don't know much about these things but when I started taking them, I found that my pain pill's span of relief was much greater. I would get 80% relief for about 2.5 hours but after taking the grape seed extract, I would get relief for 6 or more hours. If you have a Trader Joes near you they have the best price . . . 7.95 for 60 at 50mg. I take 50mg 4xday . . . if you weigh a 100 lbs take 200 mg x day. I take 400mg x day . . . when I ran out, the difference was amazing. I don't know if anyone else has tried it but I can't do without. Marty

(7) A 40 year old girlfriend who had leg numbness for about five years asked to have her blood tested for Vitamin B12 deficiency because of digestive problems. Her HMO did not want to do this test for some reason and she had to argue with the doctor to get it. It indeed came out low and Vitamin B12 injections were started. She would feel better and far less weak right after the injections but it would wear off before time for the next shots, so they kept stepping

them up for her, and she still suffered numbness. An internal medicine physician recommended a 1925 book called The **Grape** Cure Diet. She found the book at a health food store, the Green Grocer. She followed it and her numbness as well as gastro intestinal problems have so far been healed. Mc

(8) I have taken myself off all my prescribed medication (with Neuro's approval) and have been taking **Valerian** tablets three time a day and **Hops** tincture 10 drops 3 times a day. It has relieved my pain much more than medications and removed symptoms like muscle spasms, some burning and tingling. It's not THE ANSWER but it does help. If anybody tries it and it works I would love to hear about it. Good Luck! Kerry

(9) I use Alpha Lipoic Acid and **Hops Fruit** to give me about 85% relief. Dick

(10) I started taking **noni juice** Saturday September 15, 1996. Almost immediately I felt I had more energy. I was sleeping less time at night, my sleep was more restful and I had more energy during the day. I have not experienced a temperature or touch sensation in my feet for more than 15 years because of neuropathy. After taking noni juice for three days I felt coldness in my feet and I could also feel the carpet and tiles on the floors in my home. Ren

(11) I have now been taking "**Valerian**" tablets and "**Hops**", by way of a herbal tincture 3–4 times a day, for 2 and a bit weeks. I am happy to report that within 5 minutes of taking the Hops I am pain free for approximately 3 hours when the pain eases back before my next dose. My legs have stopped jumping, the burning in my feet has reduced significantly and my pins and needles have disappeared. I have gone off all manufactured drugs and my head is much clearer. I feel brighter and more able to cope

with the day. . . . The Hops burn the back of my tongue a bit but I find that if I rinse my mouth really well after taking the drops this can be minimized. I would prefer this to the pain. I take the Valerian 3 times a day on a regular basis and I am sure it is the combination of the two that is working. Jessie

(12) I reduced the neuropathy in my feet by 85% in six months taking **Hops** Fruit and Alpha Lipolic Acid three times a day. Dick

(13) I have neuropathy in my feet, legs and arms. I have started using the antioxidant **pycnogenol** at my primary care doctor's suggestion. My neurologist just kind of chuckled but I have had wonderful results. My feet are numb but there is minimal pain. You must take a mg. per pound of body weight. If you weigh 150lbs, you take 150mgs a day. I buy mine at Costco and they come in 50mg tablets. I found one man on a message board somewhere that took it and he is basically pain free. Pycnogenol is pine bark extract. I never took herbs or anything before. I was just desperate to try something. It has worked for me. Hope you will have as good results as me. Another plus is there are not any side effects. I just wanted to pass this on. Patty]

Other Supplements

1. Alpha-lipoic Acid (ALA)

ALA is a **natural antioxidant** which protects nerves from oxidative damage and inflammation. Another benefit is thought to lie in its ability to raise levels of **glutathione**, which as previously noted is an enzyme acting as a powerful antioxidant itself. Alpha-lipoic acid, some-times referred to as **thioctic acid**, also appears to **chelate** damaging free metal ions.

ALA molecules are soluble in both water and fat. This is important because as a water soluble nutrient it works inside the cell and as a fat soluble nutrient it works outside at the membrane level. A free radical thus trying to damage a nerve cell could be attacked on both sides, resulting in **dual** antioxidant protection. Another consequence of this duality is that ALA connects to and enhances the action of other water soluble antioxidants such as vitamin C and other fat soluble oxidants such as vitamin E, resulting in a strengthening of the antioxidant network.

ALA supplementation has been used to treat diabetic neuropathy in Europe for years and has been the subject of numerous European investigations which seem to validate its use for that purpose.

A study at the Heinrich-Heine University in Dusseldorf, Germany, concluded that long-term treatment with ALA induced what is known as "sprouting" or the growth of **new nerve fibers** in a **regeneration process**. According to the study, a significant reduction of pain and numbness was observed in patients treated with ALA for three weeks. Moreover, no adverse side effects were noted. A report in a 1996 issue of *Free Radical Biology and Medicine* broadly concluded ALA "may be effective in numerous neurodegenerative disorders."

A Mayo Clinic investigation, reported in a September 1997 issues of *Diabetes,* found that the administration of

alpha-lipoic acid in amounts of 20, 50 and 100 mg/kg resulted in significant **improvements of nerve conduction** in diabetic patients with PN. In fact at the end of
three months, all who were treated had lost their nerve
conduction deficit. The researchers concluded that "the
antioxidant drug [ALA] is potentially efficacious for human diabetic sensory neuropathy." Numerous other studies seem to support this view.

The amount of ALA derived from regular dietary intake is ordinarily considered insufficient to obtain significant antioxidant benefits for therapeutic purposes.
Consequently it's typically supplemented, with some
practitioners recommending a daily dose of 100 to 400 mg.
(ALA is available in tablet or capsule form without a prescription.) A report published by the Life Extension Foundation goes a good deal further and suggests a dose of
500 mg *twice* a day to treat neuropathies. It described
a three week double-blind, placebo-controlled study in
1996 in Germany involving 328 Type 2 diabetic patients
with peripheral neuropathy. The improvement rate after
19 days for those on 600 mg of ALA daily was said to have
been 82.5%. Improvement rates were tallied at 70.8% for
a part of the group taking 1200 mg daily and 65.2% for
those who had taken 100 mg daily.

(Yet another German study, reported by Richard N.
Podell, M.D., in *Health & Nutrition Breakthroughs* {No-
vember 1997}, found that ALA could restore—at least
in part—diabetic **autonomic nerve function** after just
four months of 800 mg/day treatments. At the study's end
those patients given high ALA dosages showed a statistically significant improvement in their "**sympathetic**

nervous systems" while those given placebo did not. Podell maintained that the study provided "the first clear evidence that nutritional treatment alone can reverse the course of autonomic neuropathy.")

2. Gamma Linolenic Acid (GLA)

Gamma linolenic acid is a so-called "essential fatty acid." It is normally produced by **enzyme action** in the body from **linoleic acid**, a constituent of ordinary vegetable oil. Linoleic acid and GLA are precursors of the vital **prostaglandins**. These substances are hormones vital in the regulation of a number of bodily functions such as **nerve transmission** and **pain reduction**. They also enhance **oxygen delivery** in the blood circulation system and are believed to encourage **nerve growth**.

Because most people lack the ability to produce sufficient amounts of GLA by **enzymatic action**, a number of practitioners believe it needs to be supplemented. This is said to be particularly true if any functional disorder such as PN is involved. **Borage seed oil, evening primrose oil** and **black currant oil**, available in capsules, are all considered excellent sources of GLA for this purpose. It is thought anywhere from eight to 10 weeks may be required before seeing an effect from taking one of these supplements.

In a double-blind, placebo-controlled study of a group of PN diabetic patients taking 480 mg of GLA daily (reported in *Diabetes Care*, volume 16, number 1, 1993), all who were given the nutrient were said to have experienced a gradual reversal of nerve damage and improvement in the symptoms related to their peripheral neuropathies while those on placebos gradually worsened. The researchers concluded that GLA may have helped rebuild the myelin sheath around the nerves, thus restoring proper nerve conduction.

The September 1997 issue of *Diabetes* reported that in two other placebo-controlled trials involving people with diabetic neuropathy, the use of GLA demonstrated significant benefits in "neurophysiological parameters and sensory evaluations."

In an interesting study reported by the Life Extension Foundation involving a comparison of a fatty acid derivative cousin to GLA, *ascorbyl* gamma-linolenic acid, with regular GLA, the researchers found that nerve conduction velocity—a sometimes marker of nerve health—was corrected 39.8% with the regular GLA, 87.4% with the derivative ascorbyl gamma-linolenic acid and 66.8% with GLA plus ascorbate (vitamin C).

A study reported in a 1998 issue of *Diabetologia* contends there is a marked **synergy** between GLA and ALA when mixed together. The study claims a 1.3 to 1 GLA to ALA ratio is optimal against diabetic neuropathy.

Since ascorbyl gamma-linolenic acid is not available commercially, it has been suggested by some clinicians that those with neuropathy should take 1500 mg per day of GLA and an additional 3000 mg (3 grams) of supplemental vitamin C. (I'm prompted to emphasize again that suggestions like this are not of my creation. I'm passing along this kind of information so that you can discuss it with your medical caretaker to the extent you wish to pursue a particular matter further.)

3. Acetyl-L-Carnitine (ALC)

Each type of protein in our bodies is composed of different amino acids, each tailored for a specific need. **ALC** is one which helps **move fatty acids** into and around cells. It normally is found at high levels in the muscles. It also functions to **slow aging processes** and **impede** the advance of **Alzheimer's**.

From our point of view its importance mainly lies in its **neuroprotective** and **neuroenhancing** properties. Researchers have found that peripheral nerve function in diabetes is linked to nerve **myoinositol content** and that ALC can raise the levels of myoinositol in the nerves of animals with experimentally induced diabetes. It also apparently protects the nerve membranes from free-radical damage, as evidenced in other tests involving animals.

In one study small mammals treated daily with ALC for 16 weeks showed an improvement in nerve conduction velocity. Treatments also promoted **nerve-fiber re-generation**, which was increased twofold compared with non-treated diabetic mammals.

In another study, 94 patients with peripheral neuropathy were tested at the University of Chieti, Italy, as reported in a 1995 issue of the *International Journal of Clinical Pharmacological Research*. Of these, 31 were given placebos, 31 were given 500 mg daily of **ST200** (a source of L-acetylcarnitine hydrochloride which is a form of ALC) and 32 were administered one gram of ST200 daily. In assessing pain relief the researchers concluded that the one gram daily administrations were significantly more effective than the placebos and also more effective than the lesser dosages. Further, they found that safety and tolerability were satisfactory over the entire course of the study.

Other studies have also demonstrated that ALC restores **nerve receptor densities** which decline with age (receptors are sites on cell membranes where a chemical such as a neurotransmitter can bind) and enhance the effects of "**nerve growth factor**" or NGF, dealt with in the next chapter. One of these studies was conducted by researchers at the University of Florida. In a paper published in May, 1997, "New Strategies in the Prevention and Management of Diabetes and its Complications" (*Jacksonville Medicine*, May 1997), the researchers contended that ALC may have **neurotrophic** (growth regulating) properties by stimulating the synthesis of NGF.

Dr. Robert Atkins of the Atkins Center for Complementary Medicine suggests that a reasonably healthy person simply interested in improving mental and physical performance should take 500–1000 mg of ALC daily but that for therapeutic purposes up to 1500–3000 mg may be advisable if given under the care of a physician.

4. N-Acetyl Cysteine (NAC)

NAC is a natural **sulfur-containing** nutrient found in foods and produced from the amino acid **cysteine**. It is not only a potent antioxidant itself but it rapidly metabolizes into **glutathione**, an even more powerful antioxidant.

NAC is believed able to slow the aging process in a fashion similar to ALC and play a protective role against a variety of toxic hazards such as cigarette smoke, certain herbicides and acetaminophen overdoses.

The effects of NAC treatment on nerve conduction, blood flow, maturation and regeneration have been studied in diabetic mature rats.[5] The deficits in motor conduction velocity and blood flow in these studies were said to have been largely corrected in the second month of treatment, according to a recent report entitled "Neuropathy" from the Life Extension Foundation.

It's believed that other antioxidants such as vitamin C, vitamin E and selenium enhance NAC's properties, another indication of the synergistic effects from a combination of nutrients. For general use as an antioxidant some researchers advise a daily dosage of 250 to 1200 mg. As a therapeutic agent NAC has been used at dosages as high as 1800 + mg when under a doctor's supervision.

5. Glutamine

Glutamine is an **amino acid** found in animal proteins and used to maintain **brain functioning**. It's also a precursor of **GABA**, an important neurotransmitter in

---

[5] No human studies have been found pertaining to neural aspects of NAC use. In fact it's generally true there are few human studies done on any of the nutrients covered in this chapter since important research money is reserved for patentable drugs offering the promise of big dollars for the manufacturers. To understand the benefits of less profitable, unpatentable nutrients one must rely mainly on anecdotal evidence, animal studies and hypotheses based on nutrient chemistry.

the central nervous system. Additionally, glutamine can be used by cells such as glucose for **metabolic energy**. Consequently, it's popular in athletic supplements.

Powdered glutamine is considered the best way to take this nutrient. Ten to 15 grams or so per day (about two to three teaspoons) are considered appropriate for therapeutic purposes. Some conditions, though, are said to require up to 40 grams daily. Again your doctor should be consulted when considering these megadoses.

6. Coenzyme Q10

The protein molecule **CoQ10** is found in all the cells of the body and is essential to **energy production**. It also protects the body from free radicals and enhances immune systems. In addition, it slows down the aging process.

No studies were found specifically documenting the value of CoQ10 for PN but there have been comments to that effect by various medical practitioners. Dr. David G. Williams, who writes the *Alternative* newsletter, for example, suggested in his February 1996 issue that CoQ10 may be helpful both with motor and sensory neuropathies. A 1997 study performed at the Neurology Service, Massachusetts General Hospital in Boston, involving feeding young rats with CoQ10 for one to two months concluded that "coenzyme Q10 might be useful in treating neurodegenerative diseases."

Since ordinary diets supply only a fraction of what is required, this is one nutrient which is said to particularly need supplementation, especially as a person ages. Some practitioners insist that 90 mg per day is a bare minimum and that therapeutic dosages could be in the 200–400 mg daily range.

7. SAMe (S-Adenosylmethionine)

This is a **metabolite** (a substance which metabolizes another) of the amino acid, **methionine**. **SAMe** improves the binding of neurotransmitters to their respective receptors and is also essential to **enzyme antioxidants** such as glutathione.

The principal use of SAMe seems to be as an **antidepressant**; it has been widely used in Europe for that purpose for years. A number of tests support the view that it is as effective as tricyclics such as Elavil and Tofranil, discussed earlier, in fighting depression—and without their side effects.

Reportedly SAMe has shown promise in the treatment of peripheral neuropathy. Researchers at the Metabolic Disease Center, Baylor Research Institute, in Dallas, Texas, have found that deficiencies of SAMe concentrations in the central nervous system parallel deficiencies of vitamin B12 and folate. They hypothesize that deficiencies of these nutrients may cause similar neurological and psychiatric disturbances including depression, dementia, myelopathy and peripheral neuropathy. The implication would be that as these deficiencies are corrected by nutrient supplementation the disturbances would be reduced. A study is reportedly being undertaken at Mt. Sinai Hospital to investigate methionine's effect on neuropathy.

Where SAMe is used therapeutically, administrations are said to be in the range of 400–1200 mg per day. Dr. Robert Atkins suggests dosages as high as 4000 mg daily, divided into several portions, might be necessary in some cases.

8. Dimethyl Sulfoxide (DMSO); Methyl Sulfonyl Methane (MSM)

DMSO is a paint solvent said to have unusual medicinal benefits. It's both an **antioxidant** and an **anti-inflammatory** agent. One side effect tending to hold back DMSO's use is its odor, suggestive of garlic. Fortunately it's **metabolite relative** used for the same purposes, **MSM**, is odorless. Both substances are sources of **sulfur**, a critical component of many important amino acids contained in cellular proteins.

Dr. Robert Atkins suggests that the pain relief afforded by DMSO and MLM may be achieved as a result of their **blocking conduction** in nerve fibers that transmit pain signals. Both of these substances should only be taken under the supervision of a physician.

[comments re other supplements are not to be considered medical opinions and should not be relied upon as such—always consult your doctor:

(1) I started taking [**Evening**] **primrose oil** about a month ago at the offhanded suggestion of my internist. He asked if my neurologist had put me on it. When I said no,

he said he was surprised since it was something they usually had diabetic neuropathy patients take. I am not diabetic. Anyhow, I started taking it. I really don't feel it has helped. But I'll finish the ones I have on hand. Can't hurt. Jean

(2) Nothing will make you like new. I personally have found most relief from an oral version of lidocaine called mexiletine (which was prescribed by an anesthesiologist at a pain management practice). One neurologist I consulted recommended both Vitamin E (400 USP) and **Evening Primrose Oil** capsules (don't know if they're helping or not). The people who have searched for cause undergo painful nerve biopsies and several have written in that they don't advise such a course. Hope this info is helpful. Marjorie

(3) DDI can also cause neuropathy. So can the virus itself. If neuropathy is caused by the drugs, **acetyl-l-carnitine** can help. A study was published last Spring that showed that drugs decrease the level of l-carnitine in the blood and that acetyl-l-carnitine can reverse it. I had the level tested and found it somewhat low. So I started ALC and found that it really helped. Ken

(4) My doctor has just put me on the **Acetyl-L-Carnitine**. I take two 500 mg. capsules three time a day. Along with a regular vitamin program I have also just started a B-complex stress tabs and something called TTFD (coenzyme thiamin). In addition to this I am also on B-12 injections. So far not much good has come of all this. James

(5) I have been having great results with the use of **Alpha-lipoic acid** when used with vitamins and other supplements. Jim

(6) We are the ones with the PN for about 18 to 20 years now, my husband has had 5 back surgeries which Drs. thought were the culprit for the pain in the legs, which now

we believe was the PN along. I hate to keep repeating all this information, but if you missed it before, it's hard to go back and search for it. Anyway he has had more relief this last week than he has for this long a period in a long time. Besides the magnetic inner soles, we have started **Alpha Lipoic Acid**. Been taking it for a week or 10 days. This is new in the US. You need to check it out. When we saw it on the news I came straight to the net to see what I could find. It sounds great, couldn't hurt. I even feel better. If it's in the head, it works. Anon

(7) I also 'discovered' **lipoic acid** on the web and took 600 mg/day for 3 months without any results. My neuropathy is not caused by diabetes, while all the studies are with diabetics. Marjorie

(8) In Feb.98 my feet were so bad, prickly, numb, felt red hot but not hot to touch. I would have liked to cut them off. In March I started to take Hops Fruit 150mg and **Alpha Lipoic Acid** 100 mg, three times a day, By Easter my feet were 45% better and now they are about 80 to 85% better. Don't know if it will work for you but it did for me. Dick

(9) I have been taking **MSM [Methyl Sulfonyl Methane]** now for two months and so has my husband. I now have energy, I can walk barefoot (which I have not been able to do in many years!), my back pain is gone, (I can actually stand up straight now without pain) and my husband has no pain in his hands! I have also found that my joints do not ache as they did. I am taking 3000 mgs per day and my husband is taking 1500 mgs per day. We have had no adverse side affects. We have even noticed our skin does not have the dry spots we had and the brown spots and discoloring I was getting are fading away. We have not tried the cream or crystals but have heard that they work very well also. Joan

[comments re nutrient combinations are not to be considered medical opinions and should not be relied upon as such—always consult your doctor:

(1) Dale, I've been on a **vitamin/mineral supplement** program for two years. I stopped all pain and antidepressant medications two years ago and started an exercise and vitamin program. Here's what my program consists of: A high potency **multivitamin** with **antioxidants**, **fish oil** (1000 mg) which contributes to heart and vascular health, **vitamin E** (1000 mg) which is an antioxidant and aids in maintenance of red blood cells, **calcium** with **vitamin D** (500 mg) which develops bone mass (the Vitamin D assists in the absorption of the calcium), **B-100** (B complex) which is a component in various metabolic functions, **ginkgo biloba** (60 mg) which helps to improve the circulatory flow to the hemisphere of the cerebellum, **lecithin** (437 mg) HELPS TRANSMIT NERVE IMPULSES, **chromium picolinate** (200 mg) increases insulin levels so you don't store fat as readily, **vitamin C** (1000 mg) supports the immune system, **beta carotene** (25,000 IU) which is an antioxidant rich in Vitamin A, and last but certainly not least a combination of **chondroitin** (400 mg) which helps to maintain structural integrity of joints/blood vessels and **glucosamine** (500 mg) which promotes structural integrity of joints and connective tissues. Some of these I take three or four times daily. I firmly believe that this daily program has helped in keeping my body healthy and my mental outlook positive. Fighting PN takes a lot of strength . . . a healthy body is better prepared to endure the intense pain. I also recommend that you either visit a health food store or get a good book on natural healing. I focused on vitamin/minerals that were related to my particular health problems . . . you will find ones that you can tailor to yours. Talk to the health food salespeople, almost

all are trained and certified. As always, I'll close by recommending a daily exercise program. I'm convinced that it is critical to keep those muscles from atrophying. If you don't use it, you lose it!! PN is certainly a painful disease, but it's not fatal. Good Luck! Cheers/Dotti

(2) I take 50 mg Elavil at night and 100 Zoloft in the morning, plus Darvocet as needed which I use occasionally because the combo of Elavil and Zoloft work well. I work full time in a very stressful job and sometimes take the Darvocet when I get home at night. My feet are numb now but have a lot of pain in my legs yet, also lower back and now it seems to be going into my hands. I also take a lot of nutrients such as **Vit E, Dhea, Multi, Alpha-lipoic acid, flax oil, magnesium, calcium**, etc. to give the body some good things to work with. Good luck. Joan

(3) I have been taking **Vitamin E** (400 USP), and **Evening Primrose Oil**, both at the suggestion of a neurologist at a pain clinic. At the suggestion of both an orthopod and rheumatologist, I also take a **Vitamin B supplement**. Since I also take the usual variety of drug-drugs (desipramine, clonazepan, mexiletine) it's hard to say whether the vitamins are effective. I also try to stay active, exercise, swim, ride stationary bike, all of which increase circulation and give a general sense of well-being in spite of constant burning pain in my feet. Marjorie

(4) The only Rx I take for PN is Ultram, for pain relief. My Vitamin regimen is 1 **B-Complex** daily, 3Grains **Vitamin C**, 2 **Ginkgo Biloba**, 100Mg **CO-Q10**, 400Mg **Vitamin E**, & 1 **Multi-vitamin**. My Vitamin intake results from my own research into Vitamins likely to have a positive effect on the Neurologic system...the brain in particular. I think I'm getting measurable results. When I have attacks from PN they seem to be of shorter duration. Woody

(5) I've tried vitamins and herbs and feel they have helped me. I am taking a **multi** and extra **C** and **E** plus **primrose**, **ginger**, and **echinacea**. Last year I was taking a few additional herbs, but have stopped during the summer since I have no idea what was helping and what wasn't. I plan to add them back one at a time for several weeks to see if I'm getting any result. I am very interested in what others might take. The primrose was suggested by my doctor. The others I've added as I read they help inflammation or to boost the immune system. Jean

(6) I also take the **COQ10**, with **Ginkgo Biloba**. My internist and neurologist approved it. I take a **multi**, a **C**, and an **E**, and **calcium**. I do not take extra **B vitamins** because my internist has tested to see if I am low in them, and I guess I'm not. Be careful with **B6**—it is said that too much B6 can cause neuropathy. Funny world, just as chemo is given to help with neuropathy, chemo can cause neuropathy. Pearl

(7) I am having some very good relief using a combination of vitamins, minerals, and other supplements. This includes **Alpha-Lipoic acid**, **Vitamins E, B, C,** and other products that are not toxic which are helping me to a great extent. I have cut way back on the meds, am sleeping better than I can remember, and I feel a hell of a lot better. I have been doing this for well over a month now and didn't want to give out any false hopes until I was on this program for two months. I then plan on stopping for a week and use that as a way of pinching myself to see if it is for real and, not some relapse, that I was going thru. James

(8) I too am taking some herbal supplements. Currently the only prescribed medication I am on is Glyburide. I am also taking **Evening Primrose Oil** (the only herb that has been proven to be beneficial. This was done through double-blind tests). I also take **flax seed oil, multi vita-**

mins, and enteric coated aspirin. At the moment I seem to have probably 80 percent of the pain and discomfort under control, this after suffering with a lot of pain for about 2 years. Bob

(9) I take 1 100–650 Darvocet tablet at nite plus (my own conclusion-based!) 2 **Valerian** (Health food store herb) about 30 mins. prior to the Darvocet. At lunch, with my meal, I take 2 **Vit B12** tabs; suggested by my psych. Anon

(10) I have had neuropathy for almost 2 years in my feet, and it has slowly spread toward the ankles. I tried acupuncture for a full year, almost every week, and I can't say that it was helpful. On the advice of an endocrinologist, I have been taking **Vitamin B-6** (100mg/day) for 2 years. I also have been taking **Evening Primrose Oil** (1000 mg/day) which I heard about on the Internet, from an article originated in Norway. I have been taking the Primrose oil about a year and a half. I have no idea if either the vitamin or the Primrose oil are helping me—who knows if it would be worse without them? Anon]

*   *   *

I've come to believe that, just as with exercise (discussed later), a program of nutrient supplementation can be important in dealing with peripheral neuropathy. Unfortunately, though, there seems to have been no research performed (not surprising since there's little grant money for this kind of thing) ranking specific nutrients for effectiveness. That could help us know which nutrients to concentrate on, weighing, for example, benefits versus costs among the various possibilities. (Of course it could be argued any such study would be somewhat irrelevant because of the demonstrated synergistic effect of some of these substances when taken together.)

One thing is clear: it's difficult determining what's working for you and what's not when you're taking a combination of nutrients, especially when you're likely to be taking one or more pharmaceuticals as well.

It seems nutrient selections at this time simply have to be based on information from various studies directed to specific items as well as on common sense and anecdotal reports of those who have used particular health aids. The discussions and the PNer comments in this chapter hopefully will help you in this kind of evaluation.

For whatever it's worth, *based on my own experience,* I think a regimen of antioxidants is beneficial, such as found in a good B complex along with perhaps 1000 mg of vitamin C and 400 IUs of vitamin E thrown in daily. I supplement that with folic acid (400 mcg), B12 (100 mcg), alpha lipoic acid (60 mg), evening primrose oil (1000 mg), zinc (50 mg) and selenium (50 mcg). I get other minerals such as magnesium and chromium in a daily multi-vitamin pill.

Is all that too much? Too little? I don't really know. Some part or perhaps all of these things together seems to be working for me—together with Neurontin (900 mg daily)—because most days I feel a whole lot better than a year and a half ago when starting this program.

One last note. I think if you're considering nutrient supplements you should go over your intended program with your doctor. Not only is this prudent for general safety reasons but he or she may know and be able to advise you concerning particular cautions or contraindications as they might apply specifically to you.

Chapter 7

Experimental or "Unapproved" Drugs

This chapter covers everything I could find on promising new treatments for peripheral neuropathy as well as current information concerning older experimental drugs still being considered. In fact some may think it covers too much—that PNers for the most part just want to know what's available now, not what may be two or three years in the future.

If the coverage therefore seems excessive I apologize but I feel obligated to include it all anyway. At this time we simply cannot know which new, experimental treatment might be the answer we are looking for. My sense is that *most* PNers want to know as much as possible concerning what may prove out later. I think having this information, in fact, can help us handle our present situations more easily by giving us a reason to hope that something better lies ahead.

By the time you read this, of course, some of the compounds discussed may have been dropped by investigators altogether while others may be much further along approval channels. And new compounds may well have emerged fresh from laboratories.

In spite of the fact that information here is thus inevitably dated it at least shows in which directions researchers were moving in 1999—the *kinds* of things and the mechanisms of action they were investigating which might bear fruit in the future. And, if it's not too much to hope, it might even be that sooner rather than later one or more of these compounds will either end this miserable malady of ours or so reduce its symptoms that PN becomes largely irrelevant in our lives.

The treatments are listed in alphabetical order since no other arrangement made particular sense, either by type of neuropathy addressed, benefit sought or mode of action employed. Clearly the aldose reductase inhibitors and aminoguanidine are directed at diabetic neuropathies and Peptide T is aimed at HIV-related nerve disorders. And even though most of the other compounds discussed are mainly for pain relief, classifications tend to blur with respect to benefits, etc., for compounds in the nerve regenerating group and for Bimoclomol, Nimodipine and possibly PN 401.

Aldose Reductase Inhibitors

When **blood sugars** in people with diabetes are above normal levels the body responds by channeling the excess into other sugar forms such as **sorbitol**. An accumulation of sorbitol is often found in diabetic nerve tissue where it seems to upset the chemical balance in nerve cells and increase the amount and severity of diabetic neuropathy.

The enzyme or protein which produces sorbitol in the body is called "**aldose reductase**." The overactivity of this enzyme is thought to cause neurological problems for many people with diabetes. Drugs that reduce aldose reductase activity are called **aldose reductase inhibitors** (ARIs). The result, at least in theory, is that following their administration for an appropriate period, nerve function will be maintained or restored in people with diabetes and that any peripheral neuropathy will be mitigated.

1. General Clinical Studies

In spite of this theoretical promise, ARIs have shown mixed results in PN studies over the years. In an early "meta-analysis" (a synthesis of various studies performed over a period of time), a complete search of the Cochrane Diabetes Group's database was undertaken. Results from 19 trials involving four different ARIs used to treat diabetic PN were examined. The researchers found a "small but statistically significant" improvement in *motor* **nerve conduction** velocities. No clear benefit, however, was noted in *sensory* **nerve conduction**, a principal marker in distal symmetrical polyneuropathy.

Nerve conduction velocity was also the endpoint or marker used by the "Italian Study Group" in 1996 in another meta-analysis reported in *Diabetes Medicine*. This review covered 13 randomized clinical trials published between 1981 and 1993 concerning the use of various un-specified ARIs in diabetic PN. The researchers concluded that although trials of at least one year duration indi-cated a **"significant benefit"** for motor nerve conduction velocities, no "clear conclusion about the efficacy of ARIs" could be drawn for the treatment of diabetic PN.

Also in 1996 investigators in this country made a com-prehensive review of 15 studies evaluating the effects of various ARIs on diabetic **autonomic** neuropathy and 32 studies of ARIs' effects on diabetic distal symmetrical polyneuropathy–**sensory** neuropathy. These studies had been performed over a 16-year period and involved 2511 patients. The reviewers concluded that the clinical role of ARIs is to **slow** the progression of neuropathy rather than **reverse** it. (Reported in *Diabetes*, September 1997.)

Finally a 1997 Russian study performed at the A.V. Palladin Institute of Biochemistry concluded that results there "confirmed the important role of aldose reductase inhibitors" in the **improvement** of diabetic neuropathy. So there we are—definitely a mixed bag! Nevertheless, some of the ARIs discussed below would appear to show new promise.

Incidentally, researchers at the University of Scran-ton (as reported in the book *High Speed Healing* by the editors of *Prevention* magazine) found that 500 mg of **vi-tamin C** a day in the form of a citrus juice extract re-duced sorbitol in red blood cells of diabetic volunteers by 27% and an intake of 2000 mg daily by almost half (44%)! Apparently direct linkages to nerve functioning or PN were not explored. (The possible role of bioflavonoids as ARIs was mentioned earlier in the discussion of herbs.)

2. Specific ARIs

Two ARIs which had shown earlier possibilities have been withdrawn from trials entirely. **Sorbinol** reportedly caused severe side effects in about 10% of patients taking it and **statil** simply did not prove effective. Clinicians now believe several "new" compounds merit consideration. Following, among a host of ARIs, are the ones most frequently discussed.

(a) Epalrestat

This drug was studied in 45 patients with diabetic PN at Kanazawa Medical University in Japan in 1995. The researchers claimed that subjective symptoms such as pain and numbness were "significantly relieved" after 12 and 24 weeks of treatment and that there were no adverse effects on glucose or lipid metabolism.

In another Japanese study in 1998 (at the Miyazaki Medical College) involving small mammals in which diabetic neuropathy had been induced, a significantly **greater NGF content** and **faster nerve conduction** velocities resulted from the administration of **epalrestat** according to the investigators.

(b) Tolrestat

Early studies using this ARI proved inconclusive because it was said changes in neuropathy were not measured accurately enough. Researchers in a 1995 study at the Servizio di Medicina Generale in Rome, however, concluded after a placebo controlled trial in which **tolre-stat** was administered for six months to 74 diabetic patients affected by peripheral neuropathy, that the drug produced "mild but significant" improvement. In the same year a study performed at St. Paul's Hospital, Saskatoon, Saskatchewan (reported in the July–August 1995 issue of *Annals Of Pharmacotherapy*), while generally concluding that modes of treatment of diabetic PN were unsatisfactory, found that "aldose reductase inhibitors, particularly tolrestat, have been shown to improve objective and subjective neurologic function."

Clinical studies involving 738 patients with diabetic neuropathy were described in an October 1996 issue of *Diabetes Care*. Motor nerve conduction velocities were used as endpoints for nerve function. The authors concluded that although patients treated with tolrestat had "a reduced risk for developing nerve function loss compared with placebo-treated patients," future long-term trials were needed to evaluate the impact of tolrestat treatment on "more clinically meaningful endpoints."

The future of tolrestat would still appear in doubt. Following reports of liver malfunctions from use of the drug, one of the manufacturers decided to withdraw it from foreign markets where it was being sold, ironically in the same month the above mentioned *Diabetes Care* article was published. There was a more recent problem with the drug in a study reported in the July–August 1998 issue of the *Journal of Diabetes and Its Complications*. Even though the researchers concluded that tolrestat improved autonomic nervous system function in 35 diabetic patients evaluated over a two-year period, three of the participants had to be withdrawn because of the development of "high transaminases levels."

(c) Zenarestat

This ARI which is being developed by a Japanese company, Fujisawa Pharmaceutical, is presently undergoing Phase III trials[1] in the United States. Warner-Lambert Company is a co-sponsor and will have certain rights to the drug outside the Orient. (Zenarestat is currently available commercially in Japan.)

Recently I spoke with one of the investigators who said these trials should be completed in mid-1999 and that preliminary results looked extremely promising. She also made the point that **zenarestat** is primarily designed to **protect** rather than repair nerves but that it might be used in conjunction with NGF (discussed later) for both purposes.

(d) Zopolrestat

Pfizer has developed an oral ARI, **zopolrestat** (more recently named **Alond**), which is undergoing an 18-

---

[1] Before the FDA will consider approval of a drug for marketing it must go through three testing phases. Phase I clinical trials are principally designed to examine safety. Phase II trials are designed to confirm safety and determine efficacy in humans over the short term. The purpose of Phase III trials is to prove efficacy and safety over the long term. These latter trials are usually double-blinded and placebo-controlled and can involve hundreds or even thousands of patients over many months or even years.

month multi-center trial for patients with "peripheral symmetric diabetic polyneuropathy." At the end of the 18-month period patients will be allowed to receive the drug in a continuation study. Reportedly, this drug has shown beneficial results in preliminary studies although it was suggested that "liver function changes" could result from its use. In a symposium held in June 1996 in conjunction with the annual meeting of the American Diabetes Association it was reported that zopolrestat had been shown to significantly improve nerve conduction velocity in humans after 12 weeks of treatment.

(e) FK-366

In the same symposium it was reported that **FK-366**, a "new agent," was the first ARI to decrease sorbitol levels by as much as 85%. The statement was made that "previous" ARIs were only able to decrease sorbitol by 50%.

(f) SG-210

A study reported in the May 1998 issue of the *Journal of Diabetes Complications* involved a new ARI, **SG-210**. Japanese investigators on the staff of this drug's manufacturer contend that studies of the drug in diabetic small mammals indicated it was two to five times more potent than zenarestat in suppressing sorbitol in tissues and also that epalrestat was "much less potent" than SG-210. (Corporate bias duly noted.)

Clearly, the role of specific ARIs in the treatment of

diabetic autonomic neuropathy and diabetic distal symmetrical polyneuropathy has not been secured (or as
some might say, perhaps even adequately defined). Nevertheless, efforts seems to be accelerating, as witnessed
by the brisk corporate competition noted above, to develop and test ARI compounds which might prove helpful
in dealing with these neuropathies.

Aminoguanidine (pimagedine)

Just as ARIs inhibit or retard the build-up of sorbitol,
aminoguanidine appears to inhibit or block the development of what are known as "**advanced glycation
end products**" or AGEs. High levels of these glucose-
modified proteins are frequently associated with diabetic
peripheral neuropathy.

In a number of studies involving animals, it has been
demonstrated that aminoguanidine prevented accumu-
lations of AGEs and that it increased nerve conduction
velocities. From these studies investigators at several institutions (e.g., the Department of Biomedical Studies at
the University of Aberdeen in Scotland; the Department
of Pathology and Neurology in Hirosaki University
School of Medicine in Japan; and the Department of Neurology at the Mayo Foundation in Rochester, Minnesota)
concluded that aminoguanidine may have potential in
the treatment of human diabetic neuropathy.

Alteon, Inc., has been working to develop aminoguanidine compounds in collaboration with Genentech, Inc., for
a number of diabetic applications. The company an-

nounced in late 1998 results from a "Phase III ACTION 1" trial of pimagedine (aminoguanidine) involving Type I diabetic patients with **overt nephropathy**. This is a disease of the kidneys, caused by damage to the small blood vessels, which often afflicts long-term diabetic patients. Alteon said the test data did not reach "statistical significance." Earlier pre-clinical indications had been that the compound could be helpful in dealing with diabetic *neuropathy*. Because of disappointment concerning the trial results the future of its pimagedine is in some doubt.

COX-2

There has been a race among major pharmaceutical companies to develop analgesics which relieve the pain of **osteo-** and **rheumatoid arthritis** while avoiding side effects of the non-steroidal anti-inflammatory (NSAIDs) medications usually used for this purpose. These can include stomach perforations and ulcers. Researchers believe the new pain killers may find applications in other areas, including the relief of neuropathic pain, where NSAIDs are indicated but not well tolerated.

Called **COX-2 inhibitors**, the drugs work by inhibiting an enzyme responsible for producing pain and inflammation without affecting another enzyme (**COX-1**) which primarily protects the stomach lining. The problem with the NSAIDs such as ibuprofen and naproxen is that they inhibit the beneficial COX-1 as well as the COX-2.

In two recent studies undertaken at the Kyoto University Hospital in Japan (reported in the February 1998 issue of *Neurology* and in the July 1998 issue of *Neurore-port*) the investigators concluded that COX-2 inhibitors had potential as effective therapeutic agents in "human inflammatory neuropathies."

Searle's COX-2 inhibitor, **Celebrex**, has recently been approved by the FDA to treat rheumatoid arthritis and osteo-arthritis. Merck's **Vioxx** is believed close behind. More work remains, however, to demonstrate the usefulness of these drugs for neuropathic pain.

Frogs and Snails (But No Puppy-Dogs' Tails)

The promise of ARIs and aminoguanidine lies in their ability to lessen the severity of neuropathies and increase nerve function in people with diabetes. They do this by overcoming the effects of elevated glucose levels. In a fashion somewhat similar to the nerve regeneration compounds discussed later, they treat the underlying neuropathic cause.

The two drugs in this section are targeted not at enhancing nerve function per se but rather toward **reducing** the *pain* of neuropathy. **ABT-594** and **SNX-111** are both based on chemicals occurring naturally in living creatures.

1. ABT-594

This drug is based on a poisonous substance—**epibati-dine**—secreted from the skin of the **Poison Dart Frog** which lives in tropical rain forests. The frog's name comes from the fact that natives use the poison on their arrows or darts when hunting game (and sometimes each other).

National Institute of Health researchers a few years ago found that epibatidine resembled **nicotine**, which attaches to nerve cells and produces a mild analgesic reaction. Scientists at Abbott Laboratories went a step further and identified a compound on which they had done research with a chemical structure similar to epibatidine's. That compound also attaches to nerve cells while lacking epibatidine's toxic effects.

Dubbed **ABT-594**, the new compound is said to be potentially 200 times more effective than morphine in blocking pain. Reportedly, it does this without that opioid's side effects such as addictiveness and constipation. (The sub-section "New Approaches" under "Opioids" appearing earlier dealt with other ways morphine usage might be side-stepped in the future.)

Abbott scientists, as reported in an August 1998 issue of *Brain Research,* tested their compound on two models of neuropathic pain (one diabetic) and validated, to their satisfaction, its benefits for that purpose. Safety tests are reportedly taking place in Europe at this time.

2. SNX-111 (ziconotide)

A synthetic molecule has recently been developed based on the paralyzing **neurotoxin** of a **Philippine sea snail**. According to reports, the compound, known as **SNX-111**, dramatically blocks pain in patients who no longer obtain relief from opiate drugs. It is claimed to be 1000 times more potent than morphine (which I guess would make it five times more effective than ABT-594!).

SNX-111 is considered a **calcium channel blocker**— a class of pharmaceuticals designed to block the influx of calcium ions into a cell's interior. Specifically SNX-111 is said to block **N-type**, neuron specific channels. Conventional calcium channel blockers on the other hand are said to act on the **L-type** channels found primarily in cardiac and vascular smooth muscles.

The influx of calcium ions into the interior of nerve cells triggers the release of neurotransmitters which route signals between nerves, including those which carry pain. The blocking of the calcium influx thus prevents the transmission of these pain signals. The SNX-111 molecule is said to be just the right size and shape for this purpose.

Dr. William Brose, formerly director of the pain clinic at Stanford University School of Medicine, did an early study in which SNX-111 was infused directly into the spines of seven volunteers who had suffered chronic pain for more than 35 years because of amputations or nerve damage. After three days, five of the volunteers reportedly claimed their pain had disappeared!

A division of Elan Corporation (formerly the Neurex Corporation) has been the leader in developing the compound which it re-named **ziconotide**. In late 1998 Elan reported results from a Phase III trial. Of 250 patients who were tested and who had previously failed to respond to traditional opioid therapy (some of whom had

not even received adequate relief from intraspinal morphine), 57% were reported to have experienced significant pain relief from the compound. Elan reportedly
plans on filing a New Drug Application with the FDA in
1999. It is possible that if approved this extremely
promising pain reliever could be available to PNers before the year 2000.

Lamotrigine (Lamictal)

This drug was originally developed to treat epilepsy
under the trade name **Lamictal** and has been approved
by the FDA for that purpose. The manufacturer, Glaxo
Wellcome, recently concluded a randomized, double-
blind, placebo-controlled study of 42 HIV patients with
peripheral neuropathy.

Results were presented at the eighth annual Neuroscience of HIV Infection meeting in Chicago in June
1998. Reportedly, after 14 weeks of administration, pain
was reduced significantly more for the nine patients who
had received the drug than for the 20 patients who were
given placebos. Several of the nine noted pain relief as
early as two weeks of treatment. (Five people left the
study due to rash, one due to gastrointestinal problems
and seven for non-medical reasons.)

While the precise mechanism of action has not been
determined, researchers think the drug inhibits the release of **excitatory amino acids** such as **glutamate**
and **aspartate**.

At the time this was written Glaxo Wellcome was planning a new study involving a larger number of participants.

Memantine

This analgesic, available now in Germany but not in the U.S., was developed by a small California medical company, Neurobiological Technologies, Inc. (NTI).

Memantine is a so-called **NMDA** (N-methyl-D-Aspartate) **antagonist**. NMDA receptors are embedded in the cell membranes of neurons. When activated by the neurotransmitter, **glutamate**, they open a channel through which calcium ions pass. Sometimes neurons which are damaged permit too much calcium to enter the cell, leading to further damage—a self-perpetuating state called "**excitotoxicity**." This in turn can lead to neuropathic pain under certain conditions.

NMDA antagonists such as Memantine reduce the potentially damaging influx of excessive calcium ions. Some antagonists appear to act by completely **blocking** the receptor channel. NTI claims that Merck's **MK-801** and another NMDA antagonist, **phencyclidine**, act in this fashion, preventing the normal functioning of neurons and producing undesirable side effects. In contrast, the company says that its Memantine NMDA "**modulates**" the receptor channel, eliminating these side effects.

The March 1998 issue of *Medical Sciences Bulletin* said that various studies done on rat models with chronic

nerve injury pain indicated Memantine was the most effective NMDA antagonist in relieving pain at a dose level
that did not cause motor impairment.

In January 1998 NTI announced results of a Phase II
clinical trial involving 122 patients, 60% of whom had diabetic neuropathy. The company said that after eight
weeks of treatments the patients reported on average an
18% reduction in day time pain and a 30% reduction in
nocturnal pain. In late 1998 a broader Phase IIb trial
was instituted evaluating Memantine at 22 test sites
and involving 375 diabetic patients with neuropathy.

"Natural" Pain Relievers

The body itself produces substances which can be **enhanced**, **synthesized** or **mimicked** to relieve pain. The
ones mentioned here, and their progeny, appear particularly intriguing.

1. Bimoclomol

Heat shock proteins (HSPs) are produced within the
body in response to **stress**. They are believed to be responsible for protecting the function and structure of cells.
The expression of HSPs increases rapidly not only after a
heat shock but also after various **stress** conditions.

A Hungarian company, Biorex, has developed a compound called **Bimoclomol** which artificially triggers the
production of HSPs to help injured cells **heal** them-

selves. Studies were performed (reported in a recent issue of *Brain Research Bulletin*) on small animals in which diabetic neuropathy had been induced. It was determined the compound significantly improved nerve conduction velocities. From this the investigators concluded the drug might be a useful treatment for diabetic peripheral neuropathies.

Doctors at the University of Chicago are said to agree with that assessment. In fact they reportedly believe Bimoclomol is one of a new crop of protein triggering drugs which could prove useful in treating scores of diseases.

In late 1997 Biorex entered into an agreement with Abbott Laboratories for the joint development and commercialization of Bimoclomol. Dr. Andre Pernet, heading Abbott's research efforts on the compound, told me Bimoclomol's efficacy in humans has yet to be tested. He said the objective of Phase II trials, planned in the near future, would be to determine whether the compound might slow the progression of diabetic neuropathy. There is no expectation, he added, that Bimoclomol would actually reverse a neuropathy already established.

2. Cannabinoids

There are two natural **cannabinoids** released in the body when people are injured. These are chemicals similar in structure to the crystalline phenols found in the resin of the hemp plant. This release takes place at the site of the injury with the cannabinoids acting as **filters** to control whether and what kind of a pain signal is sent to the brain.

Each cannabinoid has its own **cellular targets**—different receptors attached to sensory nerve endings. According to an article in the July 16, 1998, issue of *Nature,* one of the cannabinoids—**anandamide**—appears to attenuate immediate pain sensations while the other—**palmityethanolamide**—has longer lasting effects. When the two are administered together from external sources they seem to act synergistically, reducing pain responses more than 100 times from what would result from either given alone.

Dr. Daniele Piomelli of the Neurosciences Institute in San Diego, California, who discovered the synergistic effect of the two natural chemicals acting at the injury site, says he is working on ideas for drugs that would mimic their action.

(It might be recalled that one of the drugs discussed earlier in this book under opioid "New Approaches," is a synthetic version of a different kind of cannabinoid—one derived from the marijuana plant—with similar effects to the two "natural" cannabinoids mentioned here.)

3. Endorphins

Endorphins (together with their smaller amino acid cousins, **enkephalins**) are **neuropeptides** found in the body which are chemical messengers similar to neurotransmitters. They bind at opiate receptor sites of neurons, just as morphine does, to help alleviate pain. They also are believed to affect mood, pain perception, memory retention and learning. (For example, as mentioned before, endorphins give what some call "runner's high" following vigorous exercise.)

Laboratory experiments have shown that painful stimulation in the body leads to the **release** of endorphins. Researchers have discovered that these neuropeptides turn up in **cerebrospinal fluid**, the liquid which circulates in the spinal cord and brain. It is believed that if this fluid were fortified with additional endorphins, more nerve cells would be bound and quieted. These findings could lead to practical applications in using synthetic derivatives of endorphins for pain relief.

4. Nocistatin/OFQ2

Two more pain healers having similar characteristics might point the way to other new medications. These also are produced naturally. One, called **nocistatin**, was recently discovered by researchers at the Kansai Medical University in Japan. The second, designated **OFQ2**, was identified by scientists at the Memorial Sloan-Kettering Center in New York. The two are manufactured by the body from the same **peptides** (short proteins) and similarly act on the central nervous system by binding to cell membranes in the brain and spinal cord.

The Japanese researchers injected nocistatin (obtained from bovine brain material) into mice and found the peptide blocked the sensation of painful stimuli by seemingly counteracting another peptide in the body. This latter substance is known as **nociceptin** and has an opposite effect to nocistatin—either by amplifying pain or by turning otherwise harmless stimuli into painful sensations.

The New York team injected OFQ2 into mice and determined that their drug also blocked pain stimuli (as reported in the April 20, 1998, issue of *Neuroreport*). Related 1998 studies performed at another Japanese institution, the Nagasaki University School of Pharmaceutical Sciences (reported in *Proceedings of the National Academy of Sciences*), studied what appears to be the same protein and found that it actually triggered the perception of pain at low levels but relieved pain at high levels!

Researchers indicate that new analgesics based on nocistatin and OFQ2 could be useful in dealing with neuropathic pain, which as we PNers know is pain which often does not respond to other measures.

Nerve Regenerating Compounds

The ability of damaged nerves to renew themselves and have their functionality restored could lead to a **true cure** for peripheral neuropathy rather than just another pain reliever. Research in this area has been mainly directed towards working with "**neurotrophic factors**." These are **naturally occurring** proteins which act on neurons to support their growth and function. **Nerve growth factor** or NGF, **IGF-1** and **Neutrophin-3,** all discussed below, fall into this category. **GPI 1046**, which also appears to regenerate nerves, is a substance **syn-thesized** from a **transplant drug**.

1. NGF

NGF is a naturally occurring **protein** which helps the body produce, repair and strengthen **small** nerve fibers. The small fibers, it may be recalled, are those which carry the long lasting, aching pains many PNers experience. The identification of NGF led to a Nobel prize in 1986 but it has only been fairly recently—since cloning techniques and large scale production of manufactured or **recombinant NGF** (rhNGF) was made possible—that practical applications have been investigated.

This protein works by helping damaged neurons **grow back** toward the natural targets they are supposed to innervate—for example, muscle or skin tissue-and make precise connections there. (Following nerve damage, if the target tissue doesn't release the proper type of neurotrophic or growth factor required by the re-generating neuron in sufficient amounts, the connection will either not be made or will fail.)

Confirming its nerve growth potential, NGF has proven useful in helping **reconnect** severed nerves. Re-searchers at Duke University demonstrated in a recent study of small animals that severed motor nerves recon-nected 90% of the time when **"nerve guides"** which brought the nerve endings together were filled with NGF. This compared with a 50% success rate when NGF was not used in the guides.

Somewhat earlier studies pointed to the possible usefulness of NGF in treating peripheral neuropathy, particularly as experienced by people with diabetes. Investigations at the Neurobiology and Anesthesiology Branch at NIH in 1995, and at the University of London in 1995 and the Royal London Hospital in 1996, indicated there were significant depletions of NGF in diabetic PN subjects (both human and animal). Manifestations of **deficient neurotrophic support** were corrected by intensive **insulin** and **rhNGF** treatments.

A study led by researchers at Mayo Clinic and involving 1200 diabetic PNers was begun in 1997. RhNGF, supplied by Genentech, Inc., is being administered monthly to the test subjects. Neurologist Leland Scott at the University of Vermont College of Medicine, who is also a consulting professor at NIH, helped develop a special test-called **skin-punch biopsy,** which is being used to measure the effect of the substance on study participants and which permits the identification of **regenerating fibers**. A spokesperson at Genentech told me that results from this Phase III clinical trial[2] could be available mid-1999. (It was found quite effective in the Phase II trial.)

In June 1998, researchers evaluating recombinant

---

[2] Anyone interested in clinical trials of experimental PN drugs with access to the Internet should definitely bookmark the site: **www.centerwatch.com**. It provides information concerning ongoing trials. Center Watch even has an e-mail notification service whereby you can be informed of new trials. The main fault I find is that they do not always up-date their information so one can't tell whether a trial is currently open or not.

NGF (rhNGF) for peripheral neuropathy in another
Phase III trial, this one for HIV patients, reported preliminary results which were "somewhat mixed" (clini-
calese for disappointing). The trial lasted 18 weeks and
involved 180 subjects with PN. Doses of rhNGF supplied
by Genentech were measured at two different levels
against placebos. It was concluded that subcutaneously
injected NGF significantly reduced pain but that quanti-
tative sensory testing "did not document a return of function in peripheral nerves." The only side effect noted was
pain at the injection site.[3] The researchers stated that
"whether NGF will become a viable treatment for HIV-
PN in the future remains unclear." The latest information available from the company indicates it is not planning any further studies in the HIV population, a
disappointment to many in that group.

A small company, Cambridge NeuroScience, Inc., is
also working on NGF. The company calls its compound
Glial Growth Factor 2 (GGF2). Cambridge reportedly
demonstrated, in a study conducted in collaboration with
doctors at Albert Einstein College of Medicine in New
York, that GGF2 was effective in decreasing the severity
of multiple sclerosis by promoting the growth of new
myelin. (Similarly to some types of peripheral neuropathy, MS is a disease resulting from autoimmune attacks
on the myelin coating of nerves in the central nervous
system.) The company maintains its GGF2 should have a

---

[3] One participant noted: "The drug [recombinant NGF] cut my pain
in half during the first three months, and the pain has remained stable since. Subcutaneous injections twice per week, only side effect is
the injection site [is] black and blue for several days."

positive effect on other degenerative diseases, including diabetic PN.

A related development which could push NGF technology along faster is a recently announced collaboration between Signal Pharmaceuticals and a Japanese company, Nippon Kayaku. The two are seeking to demonstrate that a NGF **mimetic**, or synthetic molecule, developed by Nippon might be effective in dealing with damaged nerves. Signal has developed a line of **cloned** human neuronal cells which will be used to test the Japanese company's molecules "in vitro."

2. IGF-1

IGF-1 is an insulin-like **neurotrophic factor** produced by the liver and considered essential for normal growth of skin, bone and nerves. Several studies have shown that when glucose levels are high in people with diabetes, nerve cells produce less IGF-1 than normally.

Dr. Eva Feldman, Associate Professor of Neurology at the University of Michigan, has exposed nerve cells in a laboratory culture to high levels of glucose while providing IGF-1. She and her colleagues found that when IGF-1 was present the cells survived and when it was withdrawn the nerves died. She concluded that the factor "may ameliorate the signs of diabetic neuropathy."

Researchers at Cephalon, Inc., following studies in which recombinant IGF-1 was administered to small mammals, opined that the factor has "marked effects on the survival of compromised motor neurons and the maintenance of their axons and functional connections" and that it has "potential utility" for the treatment of certain neuropathies. Investigators at the Department of Neurology at the Albert Einstein College of Medicine were in agreement with that assessment, stating in a paper delivered at a 1996 symposium that pre-clinical studies suggested IGF-1 would be "useful for the treatment of mixed motor and sensory neuropathies."

More recently scientists at the University of Michigan succeeded in using IGF-1 to **regenerate** a **myelin sheath** around neurons in a culture dish. According to the researcher who presented the findings at a Society for Neuroscience meeting in New Orleans in October 1997, IGF-1 appears to be the most effective growth factor under study at "inducing myelination and preventing neural death." The findings could have particular significance for diabetic PN involving damaged myelin.

In spite of IGF-1's potential for treating neuropathies, however, a company spokesperson informed me that Cephalon is concentrating first on other possible applications such as "Lou Gehrig's" disease.

Incidentally, there is a major world-wide effort known as **The Myelin Project** (sounds like the name of a "thriller" novel) directed toward accelerating research on myelin repair. One goal is to develop an immortal line of human cells to repair myelin lesions in multiple sclerosis and in "other demyelinating diseases." The Project, headquartered in Washington, D.C., has 10 branches in various countries. Eminent researchers serve in a Work Group from such institutions as the Mayo Clinic, Yale University and the Max-Planck-Institut in Germany.

3. Neutrophin-3 (NT-3)

NT-3 is another member of the neurotrophic factor family. Pre-clinical studies of this protein (for example at the Albert Einstein College of Medicine and at the Department of Neuroscience at Genentech) have demonstrated the likely efficacy of NT-3 for **large fiber** neuropathy—the type that causes such PN sensations as numbness and tingling.

4. GPI 1046

Transplant drugs such as **cyclosporin A** and **FK 506** have the ability to enhance the growth of neuron-like cells in culture but are **immune-suppressing**. Scientists at Guilford Pharmaceuticals have been able to synthesize a new compound—**GPI 1046**—from these drugs which has **neuron-enhancing** properties but which reportedly does not have the immune suppression drawback.

Guilford's compound is an orally active **neuroimmunophilin ligand** (molecular protein) which produces nerve growth. Since it crosses the blood-brain barrier,[4] the company believes there should be no drug delivery problems. Guilford scientists have tested GPI 1046 on animals whose sciatic nerves were crushed and claim it accelerated functional nerve recovery as well as regener-

---

[4] This is a barrier membrane between circulating blood and the brain which acts as a filter to prevent damaging substances, usually large molecules, from reaching brain tissue and cerebral spinal fluid. Since neurotrophic factors are themselves typically large protein molecules, they usually cannot be administered orally or by bloodstream injection if they are to reach the brain and other components of the central nervous system where they are needed.

ated the myelin sheath. In fact the head of the company's program believes GPI 1046 has greater neurotrophic potency than nerve growth factor itself.

Guilford's president indicates the company will be actively evaluating the new drug for a number of neurological disorders such as peripheral neuropathies. It would seem, though, any useful application will be some years away; a spokesperson, who told me that pre-clinical trials of GPI 1046 were promising, indicated Phase I trials would not begin until sometime in 1999.

Guilford has granted Amgen, Inc., a much larger company, worldwide rights to develop, manufacture and sell certain of its products including GPI 1046. Considering Amgen's financial muscle and regulatory experience, the arrangement could help in bringing GPI 1046 to market somewhat more quickly if the various testing phases show positive results.

Nimodipine

This drug is another **calcium channel blocker**. It has been found helpful in treating migraine headaches although the only specific approval granted by the FDA to date is for its use in bleeding from ruptured brain aneurysms.

Early studies of **nimodipine** administered to diabetic mammals suggested that it might be beneficial in treating PN. Following these indications, a Phase I/II trial reported in the July 1998 issue of *Neurology* involving 19 patients with HIV-associated neuropathy showed "a trend toward stabilization in peripheral neuropathy." The investigators concluded that further clinical trials were warranted.

Peptide T

This is a **synthetic peptide** comprised of **eight amino acids**. It's derived from a protein of the HIV virus and has been tested on people with AIDS (PWAs) who suffer neuropathies. Press reports over the last decade seem to have raised expectations for this substance beyond its due.

Early studies did suggest the drug might be an effective pain reliever. For example, as reported in *GMHC Treatment Issues* (November 1991), the effects of Peptide T were investigated in a Canadian study involving 27 PWAs, nine of whom had PN. All reportedly experienced either complete or at least significant pain relief from injections of 10 mg per day. Beneficial effects were said to have been noticed as early as two days after treatments began. (However, two patients with numbness and sensory loss did not show improvement in *those* respects.)

Results from a double-blind study in 1996 involving 81 patients with severe HIV-related neuropathies pointed in a different direction. The study was conducted by the Department of Neurology at Mount Sinai Medical Center in New York and reported in the November 1996 issue of *Neurology*. Forty of the 81 received 6 mg per day

of Peptide T and 41 a placebo. The researchers determined that neither the change in pain scores nor nerve
conduction velocities were significantly different in the
Peptide T group as compared to the group receiving
placebos. Another study performed in Munich, Germany,
the same year had come to a similar conclusion, with the
investigators stating that Peptide T appeared to have no
effect on "neuropsychological performance or on painful
peripheral neuropathy in advanced HIV patients." (Reported in *Reuters Health Information,* July 11, 1996.*)*

Further work may be done with Peptide T for PN but
at present its future seems doubtful.

PN 401

This drug is being developed by Pro-Neuron, Inc. It is
considered a **"uridine prodrug"**—an agent ordinarily
involved in **carbohydrate metabolism**. Dr. Zachary
Simmons, Associate Professor of Medicine at Penn
State's College of Medicine, has said PN 401 "shows
great promise to improve nerve conduction for patients
with peripheral neuropathy." He is heading up one of five
study sites enrolling patients with diabetic PN for Phase
II trials.

* * *

As you may have noted, most of the studies concerning
prospective treatments have dealt with either diabetic or

with HIV-associated neuropathies. That's not surprising since, as pointed out before, these are the disorders in which big research money is being spent. Diabetic neuropathy, where the greater commercial potential lies, seems to garner more private money while HIV-associated neuropathies, where more political sensitivity exists, gets a generous helping of public funds. Unfortunately little has been done, even on a theoretical basis, to consider the implications of these compounds on the many neuropathies of other origins.

Some compounds, such as the ARIs and aminoguanidine, both dealing with excessive amounts of blood sugars and their aftermaths, may well be limited to people with diabetes even if they prove out; Peptide T (if effective with anyone) may be limited to HIV patients. But there are certainly others here, including nerve growth factors and most of the pain relievers, which would seem to be good candidates for treating diverse neuropathies. We can only hope more research in the future will be directed toward considering a wider use for these experimental drugs.

Chapter 8

Diabetes and HIV—Special Considerations

Peripheral neuropathy is frequent baggage for people with diabetes or HIV infections. Nevertheless, timely action can prevent its occurrence. Even if individuals in these high risk groups have already contracted PN, they may still be able to lessen its effects or stop its progression with proper management.

Diabetes

The American Diabetes Association (ADA) recently estimated that 15.7 million people in this country are diabetic—5.9% of the population. Of these over five million are not even aware they have diabetes! The Association also says that 65% of people with diabetes or over 10 million people sustain some kind of nerve damage. This is generally in line with other statistics which indicate that up to 50% of people with diabetes have neuropathies of varying degrees.[1] Diabetic neuropathy, in fact, is believed to represent *the most common complication* of diabetes.

Global statistics and trends give a similar picture. The World Health Organization estimates the total number of people with diabetes in the world—now at about 120 million—will double by the year 2010. This could mean there might be 120 million or more of this population with some degree of neuropathy by that time.

1. Classifications

There are **two** kinds of diabetes. The principal feature in both is the abnormally **high level of blood glucose** or blood sugar in the body. In **Type 1** (also known as insulin-dependent or **IDDM**) the elevated level is due to the pancreas not being able to produce insulin, a hormone which helps convert the glucose to energy. In **Type 2** (sometimes called non-insulin-dependent or **NIDDM** and including the vast majority of people with diabetes) the body does not effectively use whatever insulin the pancreas does produce.

Relative prevalence of the two types is influenced by **age**, **heredity** and **ethnic factors**. For example, Type 1

---

[1] The numbers vary all over the place depending on who's making the assessment. For example, in one early study, "Reported Prevalence of Symptoms and Signs of Neuropathy in Diabetics," compiled by the U.S. Dept. of Health, Education and Welfare, the reported incidence ranged from 10 to 100% of diabetic groups surveyed in four cities. The same marker, "motor conduction velocity," was used in determining the presence of neuropathy in all four cases.

is frequently diagnosed in **children** and **young adults** and often runs in families. Individuals **over the age of 45** on the other hand are more likely to contract Type 2; heredity can be a factor there also. Further, people who are **overweight** or **do not exercise** regularly are particularly susceptible to Type 2 diabetes. So are **smokers**.

Because people with Type 2 diabetes in particular often overlook or ignore the early, subtle signs of the disease, the ADA has been suggesting for years that everyone over 45 get a fasting plasma glucose test every three years. Researchers at the federal Center for Disease Control and Prevention recently have gone further. In a report published in *JAMA* in late 1998 they recommended testing begin at the age of 25.

African, Hispanic and Asian descendants living in this country are considered to be at greater risk for both types. Also it's been found that people of aboriginal descent are three to five times more likely to develop the disease than those in the general population.

2. Diabetic Neuropathy

(a) Types

The neuropathy most often affecting people with diabetes is "**distal symmetrical polyneuropathy**," a condition in which both feet and/or both hands are involved. Often this is referred to simply as **sensory neuropathy**, discussed at length earlier. Many people with diabetes also suffer **autonomic neuropathy**, which affects digestion, sweating and bladder and sexual function.

A study of 506 diabetic patients was undertaken at the Bristol Royal Infirmary in the United Kingdom several years ago (reported in the April 1995 issue of *Diabetic Medicine*) to assess the extent to which age affects the incidence of sensory as opposed to autonomic neuropathies. The researchers first determined that about half the patients in the study group had neuropathies of one type or the other. They then found that sensory neuropathy was almost three times more prevalent in those over 40 than those under 20. In contrast, autonomic neuropathy was half again more common among the group under 20 than in the other group.[2]

(b) Risk Factors

Clinicians report that diabetic neuropathy—especially that of the sensory type—usually occurs about **eight to ten years** after the onset of the disease and that the **risk** of **nerve damage** increases the **longer** the patient is diabetic. In fact an Italian study of 374 patients (reported in the March 1997 issue of *Panminerva Medica*) concluded that the **duration** of the underlying disease is the most important risk factor for diabetic neuropathy. (Taking a different view a French survey—reported in the June 1996 issue of *Drugs and Aging*—had argued that **advancing age** was a greater risk factor than duration.)

---

[2] A study reported in the April 1997 issue of *Geriatrics* concluded that diabetic autonomic neuropathy is often undiagnosed because of its "diffuse organ involvement and gradual onset."

One of the biggest problems for people with diabetes who have sensory neuropathy is their susceptibility to recurrent **foot injuries**. As is true with many of us idiopathic and other PNers, the soles of people with diabetes are insensitive to pain. This means feet can be damaged without a person even knowing it—for example by a nail or other sharp object hidden in a shoe which continues to dig into tissue. The unique problem this presents for those with diabetes, according to Dr. Anthony J. Windebank, Dean of the Medical School and Professor of Neurology at the Mayo Clinic, is that the **blood supply** to these tissues may be impaired by a diabetic deficiency of oxygen (a condition known as **ischemia**).

Dr. Windebank pointed out in the October 1998 issue of *Neuropathy News* (published by the Neuropathy Association), that this oxygen deficiency makes diabetics particularly vulnerable since ischemic tissues are easily damaged and are slow to heal. He also noted that diabetics may be more likely to develop **infections** from foot injuries because of the high glucose levels in their tissues, leading to the ultimate possibility of foot ulcers, gangrene or amputations if problems are not properly treated in time.

A common effect of **autonomic** neuropathy is a phenomenon known as **gastroparesis**, which leads to the stomach emptying its contents very slowly. This, in turn, may cause symptoms such as bloating and satiated feelings even after small meals. Autonomic neuropathy is also associated with an increased risk of diarrhea, bladder infection, impotence, dizziness and occasionally even coronary events.

(c) Blood Sugar Control

Most American investigations suggest the best thing a person with diabetes can do to prevent or lessen neuropathy, regardless of age or length of time he or she has had diabetes, is to strictly **control** the level of **blood sugar**.

Results from an important clinical study which included 1441 insulin-dependent volunteers (known as the Diabetes Control and Complications Trial) indicated that over 60% of those participants who were on an intensively managed control program for blood sugar for five years showed a lesser progression of nerve damage. Although only Type 1 diabetics were included in the study, researchers believe that Type 2 diabetics would benefit from rigorous blood sugar management as well.

Even though other studies have also reported that strict control of blood sugar **reduces pain** and **improves nerve conduction**, no one is sure exactly why. It is thought by many that glucose probably does not damage nerve cells directly but rather may affect other body systems which in turn affect the nerves. One possibility, for example, is that high glucose levels may impair blood vessels, thereby preventing oxygen and various nutrients from getting to nerve cells (the condition called ischemia as noted).

Dr. David S. H. Bell, a professor of medicine at the University of Alabama at Birmingham, had a somewhat different explanation which appeared in the June 1995 issue of *Diabetes Forecast*. He pointed out that although insulin helps glucose enter muscle and fat cells, *nerve* cells don't require insulin to take up glucose. Therefore when there's too much glucose in the blood some of the excess inevitably ends up in these cells. Once inside, the excess forms sugar alcohols such as sorbitol. The build up of these alcohols, he believes, in turn affects the production of other nutrients which the nerve cells need to function properly. After years of having to deal with this situation the nerves suffer permanent damage, according to Dr. Bell. (You may recall the earlier discussion of aldose reductase inhibitors which help limit the over-production of sorbitol. This sugar form, if not moderated, is believed to cause problems in nerve cells by upsetting their chemical balances.)

Some researchers have also focused on the effects of excessive glucose on **nitric oxide** in nerves. They point out that low levels of nitric oxide in diabetics may lead to a constriction of blood vessels supplying the nerve, thereby contributing to nerve damage.

The connection between diabetic neuropathy and nerve **myoinositol** was noted earlier. Decreased levels of inositol are frequently found in nerve cells of diabetics due to the build up of **sorbitol** in these cells caused by high blood sugar levels.

As a result of innovations such as **electronic glucose monitoring** and **insulin pumps**, blood sugar control is easier to achieve today than in the past. The ADA publishes its Buyers Guide to Diabetes Supplies in *Diabetes Forecast Magazine* every October which lists products to assist the individual with diabetes in this regard. (To order call 1-800-232-6733.)

There are also a number of drugs to control blood sugar levels which have various contraindications, side effects and methods of action. Although they do not appear to be specifically prescribed for diabetic neuropathy and thus are not dealt with here, a list would include such pharmaceuticals as **Precose**, **Glucotrol XL**, **Glucophage** and **Rezulin** (the last being the drug mentioned in an earlier footnote which reportedly had caused 33 deaths). Incidentally, according to the head of one major health plan (as reported in the November 4, 1998, issue of the *Wall Street Journal*), only about one-third of physicians who care for diabetic patients are said to employ treatments designed to keep adequate control over blood sugar levels! No documentation was given for that statement (one of my reviewing neurologists doubts it) but if it is close to being true the situation is truly appalling.

A study reported in late 1998 concerning strict blood sugar control, while not directed to diabetic neuropathy, was interesting in revealing other benefits. Of the 600 patients involved, 400 were on a special diet while taking Glucotrol XL. The remaining 200 patients were on the diet alone. After 12 weeks the patients who were on **both** the drug and diet regimen had much **better control** over blood sugar levels than the others—a result not too startling. What was noteworthy, though, was the degree to which those in that group had **more energy** and a greater sense of **well-being** than those on diets alone. In fact those in the latter group were nearly five times more likely to be absent from work than the drug-and-dieters.

(d) Other Treatment Approaches

As far as drugs targeted directly to diabetic neuropathy are concerned, the preceding chapter dealt with experimental compounds such as aldose reductase inhibitors, meant to control sorbitol, and aminoguanidine, intended to block or inhibit "advanced glycation endproducts."

Practitioners with the University of Florida College of Medicine indicate they also have had success with **Octeocide**—a synthetic substitute for a naturally-occurring hormone—in treating certain autonomic neuropathic dysfunctions affecting diabetics.

Of course a number of the drugs covered in Chapter 3 are being regularly prescribed by doctors to lessen the pain of diabetic neuropathy. Also various nutrients such as alpha-lipoic acid, gamma linolenic acid and acetyl-l-carnitine as well as the vitamin and mineral regimens discussed earlier are being used, reportedly to good effect.

Dr. Ward Dean, in his paper on "Peripheral Neuropathy" (mentioned before as the author of *Smart Drugs and Nutrients*), points out the particular benefits of **gamma linolenic** (GLA) supplementation for diabetic patients. He suggests that diabetics may have an impaired ability to convert linoleic acid to GLA, which can lead to defective nerve function.

Special mention should also be made of **inositol**, **biotin** and **thiamin** for diabetic PN. Dr. Stanley Mirski reportedly has found a large percentage of his diabetic neuropathy patients making significant improvements with daily supplementations of 50–100 mg of thiamin or vitamin B1, as have other doctors.

In addition to the various medical and alternative therapies available in dealing with diabetic neuropathy, most practitioners will generally stress the importance of **diet**, **exercise**, **weight reduction** and **abstention from tobacco**. However some doctors urge that the diabetes be brought under control first before an intensive exercise program is initiated.

The Columbia Health Corporation in a paper, "Diabetes & Exercise," makes the point that exercise *usually* lowers blood glucose levels and permits muscle cells to take in glucose more efficiently. The authors point out, though, that when glucose levels are already high (over 250 mg/dl) exercise may in fact *increase* blood sugar levels, particularly in Type 1 diabetics, indicating an insulin insufficiency. They add that in most Type 2 patients, on the other hand, high blood sugars represent insulin resistance rather than insufficiency and that exercise for these may help in reducing this resistance and lower elevated blood sugars. They urge in any event that diabetics discuss their plans with their physicians before embarking on exercise programs, particularly if a condition such as peripheral neuropathy exists.

A recent article in the *Canadian Journal of Diabetes Care* (22 [4]:39–46, 1998) warns that patients with **autonomic diabetic neuropathy** in particular should maintain proper fluid and electrolyte balance during exercise because of defects in thermoregulation, sweating and in their responses to dehydration.

HIV/AIDS

The World Health Organization reports there are about 33 million people living with HIV/AIDS. New HIV infections were estimated at 5.8 million in 1998. WHO puts the North American figure (for 1997) at 860,000, with 44,000 new cases.

About half of all people infected with HIV, the virus that causes AIDS, develop neurological complications of one kind or another, according to the National Institute of Allergy and Infectious Diseases. By far the most prevalent of these is peripheral neuropathy, believed to affect up to 35% or as many as 300,000 in North America. (The figure given at a mid-1998 Neuroscience of HIV Infection meeting for just the United States was upwards of 180,000 PN victims.)

A special problem is said to exist with respect to HIV neurological complications: many infected people have more than one disorder with overlapping symptomatic features. This makes precise diagnoses difficult and sometimes necessitates special diagnostic procedures such as **brain scans**, **magnetic resonance imaging** (MRIs) or **brain** and **spinal fluid** analysis.

1. Types

The most common type of neuropathy associated with HIV occurs generally in the later stages of the disease and is what again is referred to as **distal symmetrical polyneuropathy** (DSP), or **sensory neuropathy**. In fact a study reported in the January 1999 issue of *Archives of Neurology* found that 38% of the 251 HIV-infected individuals examined had DSP and that DSP represented the most frequent neurological disorder found in the group.

In their study, "Peripheral Neuropathies in Human Immunodeficiency Virus Infection," by David R. Cornblath et al. (appearing in the treatise *Peripheral Neuropathy*, Dyck & Thomas, W. B. Saunders, 1993), the authors reported a study of 56 patients with the "full spectrum of HIV-1 disease." Neuropathy was found in 89% of the patients. In fact, according to a paper appearing in the February 1994 issue of *AIDS Clinical Care*, autopsy-based studies have indicated nearly all patients who die of AIDS had previously suffered sensory neuropathy.

Other neuropathies frequently reported in HIV cases are **toxic** neuropathies, caused by antiretroviral[3] or so-called nucleoside analogue agents such as **ddC** (Zalcitabine) (said to be the worst of the lot), **ddI** (Didanosine) and **d4T** (Stavudine). **Isoniazid**, used to treat tuberculosis, **Vincristine**, used for Kaposi's sarcoma, and **Cisplatin** and **Taxol** (prescribed for cancers), can all cause PN as well. Clinicians believe these toxic agents do their harm by damaging **axons**—the fibrous extensions of nerve cells which communicate with muscles, tissues and organs.

Reportedly anywhere from 7 to 15% of PWAs (persons

---

[3] An antiretroviral drug is any pharmaceutical that stops or suppresses the reproduction of HIV or another retrovirus.

with AIDS) on antiretroviral treatments will develop toxic neuropathies over time. As more and more PWAs have access to such drugs and live longer it can be expected that the actual numbers will increase exponentially.

The symptoms of toxic neuropathies are similar to sensory neuropathies—burning, tingling, aching pains in the feet, and sometimes in the hands, accompanied frequently by exquisite tenderness in the distal members. Occasionally the use of one of the toxic agents mentioned may intensify symptoms of an already existing neuropathy rather than inducing one itself.

A less common but more severe disorder sometimes affecting AIDS/HIV victims is **chronic inflammatory demyelinating polyneuropathy** or CIDP, which was discussed in Chapter 4. This disorder results from damage to the fatty membrane or myelin sheath covering the nerve fibers. It is usually **autoimmune** in origin—similar to Guillain-Barre syndrome—and tends to develop relatively early in the course of HIV infections.

CIDP is characterized by a slow progression of **muscle weakness** and **loss** of **muscle control**. Often the weakness begins in the feet and ankles, leading to a clumsiness when the victim is walking, or to a slow, stumbling gait. Not infrequently a victim's ankle will give way, which can cause serious injuries.

2. Treatment Approaches

Most of the medications and therapies which work for other PNers should work for the neuropathic problems of

PWAs and HIV-infected individuals since at least some of the mechanisms are believed to be the same. Generally clinicians think the addition of a good vitamin B complex could be particularly helpful in PWA/HIV cases, noting a tendency for these patients to be especially **deficient** in **vitamin B12**.

A cautionary note has been cited by practitioners concerning the use of **tricyclic antidepressants** such as Elavil (amitriptyline) and Norpramin (desipramine) with patients who have **HIV dementia**. They say these drugs could precipitate **acute delirium** in certain cases.

One new drug currently under investigation which might prove particularly helpful in relieving pain from HIV or AIDS-associated neuropathies is **Lamictal** (lamotrigine). PWAs who received the drug in a small study reported a significant reduction in pain and tingling according to results presented at the eighth annual Neuroscience of HIV Infection meeting in Chicago in June 1998. (See the fuller discussion on Lamictal in the previous chapter.)

If the neuropathy is toxic in nature it will usually disappear six to eight weeks after the patient ceases taking the causative agent, according to practitioners. (Unfortunately some toxic neuropathies reportedly are permanent regardless of elimination of the causative agent.) It is not uncommon, in the meanwhile, for the neuropathy to worsen for a period before it is resolved—a phenomenon known as "coasting." But take note: physicians say even a limited resumption of the agent thereafter might bring the neuropathy back in full force!

Some studies have suggested that since **acetyl-l-carnitine deficiencies** have been found in PWAs who developed toxic neuropathies while on treatments with ddI, ddC or d4T, supplements of ALC should be helpful. Also researchers have noted that **magnesium deficiencies** in the nervous system can result in the accumulation of damaging toxic chemicals. It has been suggested that taking an extra 400 milligrams of magnesium a day will prevent further damage. (See the previous discussion on this mineral.)

Dr. Jon D. Kaiser, author of *Immune Power* (St. Martin's Press, 1993) and a physician at the Wellness Center in San Francisco, California, recommends anyone taking d4T also take two capsules (250 mg) of magnesium in the A.M., two capsules (300 mg) of calcium in the P.M. and one capsule (100 mg) of vitamin B6 twice a day as a preventative measure against PN. (In the view of many neurologists 200 mg per day is the upper limit for safe usage of vitamin B6.)

As stated before, most practitioners say that CIDP patients respond well to **prednisone, plasmapheresis** or **IVIg** treatments. Other approaches in these cases have involved such drugs as **cyclosporine A**, **azathioprine** and **cyclophosphamide**.

Patients with HIV infections are noted experimenters with alternative therapies. In fact various studies have estimated that up to 70% of such patients are using alternative or complementary treatments, sometimes by themselves but usually as adjuncts to more conventional approaches. Certainly one of the "most alternative" has to be the following concoction to be taken daily. It originally appeared in *Positive Health News* and was reported to reverse the effects of neuropathy in PWAs within 10 days. (No guarantees from here, though):

1. Cut one medium lemon into quarters and place in a blender together with the rind and seeds.
2. Add 1 ½ cup of orange or other fruit juice.
3. Also add one tablespoon of cold pressed Extra Virgin Olive Oil to the drink three times a week if liver bile production is normal. (If bile levels are high skip this; if low add every day.)
4. Blend at high speed for two minutes.
5. Pour mixture through a strainer to separate the juice from the pulp. Discard the pulp.

Author's note: Nobody said it was supposed to taste good. At least the last step is a relief. Anyway, skoal!

Chapter 9

Coping

It may not be possible for us to feel like we once did before we got stuck with this atrocious ailment—at least not yet, not until some true cure comes along—but there is much we can do now to improve the quality of our lives. That's what this chapter is about.

Exercise

1. Benefits

Most clinicians think the benefits of **exercise** stem largely from the **improvement** in **blood circulation** it produces. This improvement permits **oxygen** to be carried to various parts of the body (including nerve tissue) where it's needed most. Also a good exercise program will almost inevitably lead to a **loss of weight**—a desirable goal in itself for most people and one which is believed especially important for people with neuropathy. In any event as one PNer said plaintively: "At least one good thing about weight reduction is there is less of you to hurt."

Of course beyond any particular PN benefits there are a number of general health boons from exercise. These include the **reduction** of **low density lipids** (LDLs) and **triglycerides**, the **increase** of favored **high density lipids** (HDLs) and the **lowering** of **blood pressure**. David C. Nieman, professor of health and exercise science at Appalachian State University in Boone, North Carolina, also points out that moderate daily exercise can **boost** the body's **immune system**.

I found one formal study on the value of exercise to PNers. As reported in the October 1997 issue of *Physical Therapy*, 28 subjects with peripheral neuropathy between the ages of 23 to 84 were followed through a six week period during which half completed a home exercise program. Dr. Richard K. Shields, a professor in the Physical Therapy Graduate Program at the College of Medicine, University of Iowa, was the principal investigator in the study.

Subjects were given stretching bands to exercise the upper body, gradually increasing resistance, with a goal of 10 daily repetitions. They also were instructed to exercise aerobically up to 20 minutes each day, either by walking or bicycling, with enough intensity to achieve a heart rate of 60 to 70% of their estimated maximum heart rate (220 minus their age).

Study conclusions were based on impairment measures which included average muscle scores, handgrip force, walking time and "forced vital capacity." A health survey was also used which dealt with quality of life perceptions.

At the end of the six-week period those in the exercise group showed moderate improvements in their strength impairment measures, as could be expected. What was noteworthy were the significant improvements reported in the **quality of life** surveys. Exercise participants indicated on average a meaningful change in "physical and mental role limitations" (self-perceptions of physical and mental disabilities) and "social function limitations" (self-perceptions of interference with normal social activities). The study did not, however, demonstrate any overall pain reduction for those participants.[1] From an analysis of the results Dr. Shields concluded that a home exercise program should be an important component of treating people with peripheral neuropathy.

I think the message from this study is that, apart from any direct physical benefits (which can be significant), exercise makes us feel better about ourselves, that perhaps we figure we are not quite as hobbled by our PN as we previously thought, that we look better, have more energy, are generally healthier and happier, etc.

2. Types of Exercise

Of the various forms of exercise, most PNers seem to agree **water aerobics** (such as running in deep water while wearing flotation devices) or simply swimming

---

[1] One PNer got it right, I think, with this observation:

> "I didn't go into the exercise routine hoping to find a solution for my PN pain or the progression of the disease. . . . I just wanted to keep from winding up in a wheel chair. Perhaps the most benefit I get from it is that I know I am doing something good for myself. I wasted away for a couple of years in the beginning, so just knowing I'm on the positive end of the disease makes me feel good."

laps, or a combination of the two, is best since it takes the **weight off** of painful feet while you're exercising. Also it's easier to **stretch** and **work muscles** in the water. If you prefer to exercise in the shallower end of a pool you might consider buying a pair of water shoes to give your feet some protection and traction. (Occasionally people simply use old tennis shoes for this purpose.) To get the full benefit of any water workout it's suggested you spend at least 30 minutes in a pool, daily if possible but at least several times a week.

If our feet can handle **walking**—the faster the better—that also is an excellent form of exercise. Unfortunately, running or jogging must remain a memory for most of us who used to enjoy those pursuits. A **treadmill** provides much the same walking experience but under controlled conditions. (I used to have one but my feet couldn't take it anymore.)

The **Stair Master** is a step removed (no pun intended) from walking. This machine eliminates the foot impact of walking—though it can still put stress on your feet as you push down. I personally prefer a machine called the **Precor**, where you slide your legs back and forth in a gliding motion while your feet are planted on "skis." With the Precor you can increase the resistance or raise or lower the height of the ski tips on the control panel. Another so-called elliptical machine is the **Body Trek** which involves the use of arms as well as legs.

Easier on the feet yet are **exercise bikes**. A type many favor, me included, are **recumbent** models where you plop yourself in a "chair" and pedal while sitting back with your legs pumping horizontally. You can read, watch TV or just listen to music, all while getting a great workout.

Many PNers also use **strength-building** routines such as weight lifting. Well equipped fitness centers offer all kinds of equipment for this purpose.

Physical therapy experts maintain that gradual **stretching** and **strengthening exercises** help relieve the stress of chronic pain. An organization called Stretching, Inc., has a web site (www.stretching.com) offering various helpful books on stretching and body building techniques. You may also wish to look back on the section, "Physical Therapy," in Chapter 5. Incidentally, it is always a good idea to have a trained physical therapist formulate your exercise program.

One other form of exercise some PNers use, also previously mentioned (in the discussion of qigong), is the Chinese martial arts routine called **tai chi**. This is a training exercise involving slow, graceful movements such as seen performed in Chinese parks early in the morning. These movements are derived from the movements of animals and follow a natural, relaxed pattern. They increase the body's motion range and are said to exercise the internal organs. (Don't ask me how.) According to practitioners the slow meditative routine aids relaxation, stress reduction, balance and posture, and increases blood flow.

Diabetic PNers are again reminded of the cautions mentioned in the preceding chapter prior to their engaging in exercise programs.

Temperature Effects

A line from an old song, "Some like it hot, some like it cold . . . ," fits here. There are people with peripheral neuropathy who can not imagine putting their already burning feet into a pan of warm water. Others find gratifying relief from a warm soak. Then there are PNers who yearn for an ice pack, a cold compress or even a bag of frozen peas to put on their skin when things get tough and their nerves become angry.

1. Cold or Heat?

As to which is best in general—cold or heat—one can only say **use whatever works** for you. There are *some* rules of thumb, though. **Heat** generally **relieves sore muscles. Cold** on the other hand **lessens pain sensations** by **numbing** the affected area. Some think cold relieves pain faster with the relief lasting longer.

One expert on hydrotherapy claims that heated water stimulates your immune system and causes the white blood cells to move into your tissues where they help eliminate toxins and wastes. He says that cold water discourages inflammation by contracting or tightening blood vessels. He also mentions that **contrast therapies** are sometimes used where a patient goes back and forth between heated and cold water.

Chronic Pain Workbook authors Dr. Kimeron Hardin and Ellen Catalano say that both cold and heat therapy decrease the number of pain impulses sent to the spinal cord and that there is a lesser ability for the pain messages to open the pain gate.

I suppose if you were going to take a survey of PNers who use either cold or heat to at least temporarily allay their symptoms, you would find more leaning to cold. No matter which way you go though, be careful. Excessive heat or cold over numbed areas may not be noticed at first but they can cause serious harm to your skin. Therapists advise testing the temperature first and not prolonging any cold or heat treatment for more than twenty minutes.

2. Mechanisms

There are many ways to use heat for pain relief. A **heating pad** is always a good solution so long as you don't go to sleep with it on and burn yourself. **Gel packs** heated in hot water, **hot water bottles**, **heated moist towels** and simply a **hot bath** or **shower** all work well. **Heated pools** are fine too. (A physical therapy group I went to for a period had a whirlpool with the temperature maintained at 95 degrees. I would put my feet in there for 10 minutes or so while doing stretching exercises. My feet and I both felt good afterwards and we were friends once again but it didn't last long.) Infrared radiation has also been mentioned by some as a means of introducing therapeutic heat into body tissues for pain relief (but check with an expert before trying this one!).

For cold you can try **gel packs** wrapped in towels

which maintain their flexibility at freezing temperatures. Also **crushed** or **cubed ice** in towels can be used. (You need something between the ice pack or the ice and your skin so you don't get "freezer burn.") Of course there's always that **pan** or tub of **cool water** you can put your flaming feet or fiery fingers into for a few minutes of blessed relief. (Yet I remember one time doing some body surfing in the cold Pacific off La Jolla, California, and my feet began to hurt so much—the rest of me felt fine—I had to get out of the water. I never had a problem like that before I had PN.)

Sometimes when pain is so severe that it's difficult to sleep you might try putting your feet in a pan first and then slowly adding water at room temperature. Let the water keep running after the pan is filled (direct the overflow into a drain, of course, or others will be unhappy with you) while the temperature is lowered. Hopefully the water will become cold enough that most of the pain will have disappeared after five or ten minutes. Then dry your feet (maybe using a fan over them for a few moments first), hurry back to bed and try to go to sleep before the pain returns. One PNer said it's like a game sometimes—who's going to win tonight, me or my feet?

Mini Jacuzzis for your feet are on the market—small basins really in which water is squirted through jets and can be temperature controlled. I tried one model a few times but didn't get much benefit from it. I thought the idea behind it was good but mine didn't have sufficient power to make the water move enough. I think the unit is quietly resting in our attic now.

Sleeping

One only has to read comments on Internet bulletin boards and forums to see what a desperate problem **sleep** can be for some PNers. One big reason is their **super-sensitivity** to anything brushing against their feet. This makes sheets, bedcovers and even just turning over in bed at night an extremely unpleasant experience for those whose sensory neuropathy is particularly acute.

A variety of things have been tried by a number of these PNers to keep them from being unnecessarily re-minded their feet are still there, larger than life and throbbing away, as they ease into their beds. Some have built **frames** at the bottom of their beds, or purchased **hoops**, draping the sheets and covers over these devices so their feet aren't touched. Others wear **socks** and pull the bedclothes up slightly on the theory that having your feet completely covered is better than having something rub against them through the night. Others apply an **ointment** before donning the socks.

PNers have various ideas on creating the most **con-ducive conditions** for sleep. It's suggested that you should keep the room temperature around **70 degrees**, **eliminate** all **light**, get a **"white noise" device** or **ear plugs** to get rid of background noises, and learn **relax-**

ation techniques (described earlier) to go back to sleep if you're awakened.

Experts offer a number of ideas for sleep problems. The following hints are from the National Sleep Foundation (see, there's a foundation for just about everything):

1. Exercise regularly but do so several hours before bedtime.[2]
2. Avoid alcohol, caffeine and nicotine in the evening.
3. Don't nap during the day.
4. Try and follow a regular sleep schedule, even on weekends.
5. Don't use your bed for anything other than sleep or sex. The Association adds that "your bed should be associated with sleep." (No advice given on the other activity.)

Here are more tips from other experts:

1. When you can't sleep get up and do something really boring. You might try reading the warranty on the refrigerator.

---

[2] A 1997 Stanford University study indicated that people over 50— those most likely to have trouble sleeping—did better if they exercised regularly. A number of men and women were put on 30 to 40 minute exercise sessions four times a week (stationary cycling or brisk walking). Compared to a sedentary control group those in the exercise program reported they not only slept an hour longer but they fell asleep in half the time.

2. If you just can't make it through the day without a nap make the nap less than an hour and take it before 3 P.M.
3. Get up the same time every morning.
4. Have a *light* snack before going to bed. (Dairy products and turkey both contain tryptophan, said to be a natural sleep inducer.)
5. Take a hot bath 90 minutes before bedtime. The theory here is that a hot bath will raise your body temperature and then the subsequent drop will make you sleepy. (According to a study reported in the December 1998 issue of *Reader's Digest*, nine women with insomnia took a hot bath one and a half hours before bedtime for two consecutive nights and in the following week took lukewarm baths for the same periods. The women were said to have experienced a deeper and more restful sleep following the hot bath than after the lukewarm one.)

Restless Legs Syndrome is a sleep disorder related to some neuropathies in which a person experiences unpleasant leg sensations such as creeping, crawling and tingling feelings through the night. Many with **RLS** also have **PLMS** [periodic limb movements in sleep], a particularly unwelcome PN-associated disorder characterized by involuntary jerking every 10 to 60 seconds.

A study in the *Mayo Clinic Proceedings*, as reported in the February 1999, *John Hopkins Medical Letter*, found that 15 RLS patients who had not responded to other drugs experienced significant improvements in their symptoms from a new anti-Parkinson medication, **pramipexole** (trade name, **Mirapex**), after a 2 to 3 month trial period.

Foods and Diet

Much has already been written by others concerning healthy foods. Moreover, there are many books full of diet ideas on how to lose weight which would help PNers just like everyone else. Additionally, there is a great deal of specific information available concerning the **foods** diabetic PNers should **avoid** in order to control their blood sugar levels. I'll just note here a few things I've come across concerning direct linkages between foods and peripheral neuropathy:

Dr. Donald A. Twogood, author of *How to Rid Your Body of Pain*, suggests that we who have peripheral neuropathy eliminate the following from our diets. He lists them in the order of worst first. (I'm not necessarily advocating but just reporting this.):

1. Casein-based products such as milk and other dairy foods as well asnon-dairy foods such as creamers, Cool Whip and many soy milks. (Note that in the tips on sleeping just referred to, another expert **suggested** a dairy product snack before bedtime. So the big question is: who ya gonna believe?)

2. Chocolate (Interestingly the *British Medical Journal* recently reported that 7841 Harvard male graduates who ate chocolate lived a year longer on average than their non-chocolate counterparts, the speculation being that antioxidants in the chocolate made the difference!)

3. MSG (monosodium glutamate) in processed meats, packaged foods, etc.

4. Aspartame, such as found in diet sodas and in the sweeteners Equal and NutraSweet. (He has company on this one. Dr. Yngve Bersvendsen, of Bergen, Norway, in his paper, "A Multidisciplinary Approach to Diabetic Neuropathy," also urges the complete elimination of aspartame from diets.)

Others have suggested **eliminating red meats** and **refined sugar** and switching to a **vegetarian diet** as much as possible. A study at the Weimar Institute reported in the *American Journal of Clinical Nutrition* (September 1988), claimed that neuropathy symptoms were entirely relieved in 17 of 21 patients placed on a vegetarian diet and exercise. The report said improvement was noticed in four days in some patients.

Dr. Lark Lands, in her book, *Positively Well: Living With HIV as a Chronic, Manageable Survival Disease*, mentioned the University of Alabama study on the nutrient **inositol** discussed earlier in this book. Researchers in Alabama suggested PN diets favoring high-inositol foods such as cantaloupe, peanuts, grapefruit and whole grains.

The column, "The Doctor and The Dietitian," written by Dr. Ross A. Hauser (an M.D. with an avowed natural healing bent), encourages those with peripheral neuropathy to eat three servings each of **fruits** and **vegetables** daily.

For a final "hot" food idea relating to calming neuropathic pain when it gets really bad you might try the **Datil pepper**. This is a fiery cousin of the habanero pepper and is sure (just like capsaicin) to release a lot of the body's natural pain killers—if your mouth can take the heat.

Special Considerations—Feet

How to cover and protect our feet is a subject about which PNers like to talk at length—even if they have short feet. That's probably where most of us experience the worst pains.

1. Shoes

It's generally agreed that PNer shoes should be **well-cushioned**; those with air support are favored by many. Shoes made from **soft materials** which "breathe" are considered desirable. Also they should be **plenty wide** and allow the toes to **move** around **freely**. (After years of PN, **reflexes** may be lost and feet tend to become wider and flatter.) Besides the extra width may be necessary to accommodate inserts, which will be covered next.

Some prefer shoes easy to slip on. Sandals fit the bill

for this better than regular shoes. (I personally like what are called boat or canvas deck slip-ons.) A few PNers extol the virtues of wearing light-weight shoes because of their weakened foot and ankle muscles.

A dozen of the shoes PNers seem to especially favor, with some of their comments, follow. The first six are basically for women, the last six for men:

- sheepskin-lined boots called Uggs ("too sloppy for walking but great around the house")
- soft suede sandals called "Fits by Theresa" made with wide Velcro straps easily loosened or tightened over the upper foot ("expensive—I paid $128 for them but the comfort is indescribable")
- Birkenstock sandals made with deep heel cups to absorb shocks and lightweight but firm soles ("good old Birkenstocks, winter and summer, are my greatest relief")
- "Colorado" brand, styled as a closed, boxy toe sandal ("they have cork and rubber for cush, toe bumps—this helps my balance, high arches and heel cradles")
- Skechers, a casual shoe "targeted at Generation X" ("they have a huge toe box. . . . they're heavy but very stable")
- SAS "Freetimes" for women ("you can take out the liner and put in an insert . . . they really are wonderful")
- SAS "Time Outs" for men (I own a pair myself and they're great for longer walks—they have firm soles, a wide toe box and come in a variety of widths)

- Etonic sneakers ("they have a wider toe box")
- Ecco shoes ("great, but not as good as not having any shoes")
- Ahh Keds ("an upgrade from the old canvas sneaker with a removable cushioned insole")
- Nike Air Max running shoes ("I read that running not walking shoes are best . . . these are terrific")
- Rockports ("the only ones I've found that allow me to walk past the pain and get 45 minutes of exercise in 3–4 times a week")

There are also companies offering **therapeutic shoes**. They seem to cater mainly to diabetics who can receive partial reimbursement from Medicare if they have a doctor's prescription.

I came across an advertisement for **Shiatsu Massage Slippers** which looked interesting. These are made of suede and feature raised nodes which are supposed to provide a relaxing foot massage. Each slipper has an on/off button and operates on AA batteries, according to the marketer, the Innovation Shop. The regular price is supposedly $49.95 but they were available at the time this was written for $24.95 (1-888-427-7652). I have not tried them so I can't vouch for how they perform. (A few months ago I bought a battery operated, lambs-wool covered, foot massage device for about $20. It not only massaged but provided heat. Tried it once—it didn't work for me—and my wife gave it to a non-PNer friend who really enjoys it.)

Wal-Mart offers **thermal slippers** in their pharmacy sections which are made by the R.G. Barry Corporation.

You heat them in a microwave oven for a warm-up before putting them on. (Remember they're not to eat!) They are called Lava Booties and sell for about $20 a pair.

2. Inserts

There are several kinds of shoe inserts: **orthotics**, **"orthotic-type" inserts** and **cushion pads** of various configurations.

Orthotics are removable **innersoles** designed to provide support for the foot and correct abnormalities of the foot structure. Proponents say this latter purpose is particularly important for those with bio-mechanical arch problems since the rest of the body can be affected.

Orthotics are usually custom made, either as prescribed by a podiatrist or pedorthist (there are those professionals too) or created from foot impressions sent directly to the manufacturer by the user. In either case plaster foot casts are first made from impressions and then the orthotic is molded over the cast. Plastic or other material may be used for the purpose.

A somewhat similar insert is offered by the Featherspring International Corporation. They're made from spring steel and formed to foot impressions which prospective users make and send to the factory. Feathersprings don't sound particularly comfortable to me but they've had rave reviews (according to the company's sales literature) and some PNers seem to have been pleased with them. They're expensive—$220 a pair—but

Featherspring offers a 60 day trial with money-back guarantee (1-206-545-8585). (Maybe it's an "if all else fails" kind of thing for us.)

Some PNers reject the idea and expense of any custom orthotics and rely solely on other kinds of inserts which serve similar functions. Frankly I'm in that camp. Over the years I've purchased a couple sets of rigid, custom orthotic inserts, one made of hard plastic and the other leather, and found them both uncomfortable and not very helpful. I do have a foot pronation problem, though, which needs to be addressed. Two years ago an orthopedist in La Jolla, California, sold me a pair of sponge plastic molded inserts designed to support the arch which are great. Not only do they help my pronation but because they're shock absorbent my PN foot pains are lessened if I'm doing much walking. Most medical supply stores sell similar devices made of rubber or other flexible substances in the $10 to $25 price range.

I found I was not alone in thinking over-the-counter shoe inserts work just as well as custom-fitted orthotics. *Better Homes and Gardens* magazine ran an article (in January 1998) citing a study of 240 patients with heel pains in which more of them found relief from inexpensive inserts than from custom orthotics costing many times as much!

(It probably makes sense, however, for any PNer with foot problems to see a podiatrist, pedorthist or orthopedist to determine if there is a bio-mechanical condition contributing to foot discomfort before buying inserts.)

If simply getting more cushioning in your shoes against impacts is the goal **Dr. Scholl foot pads** seem to be the number one choice of most PNers—particularly the plain vanilla, single-layer, foam cushion types. They get my vote too. Occasionally I wear them along with the other inserts I use (in shoes which are cut wide and deep enough). You can keep a supply of the Dr. Scholl pads on hand—they're not very expensive—and add one or more to whatever shoes you want to wear.

Some PNers swear to the benefits of **magnetic shoe inserts**—gel or rubber insoles in which tiny magnets have been imbedded. Others object to them because they think they can feel the magnets as they walk. I've tried magnetic inserts, as mentioned before, and didn't get any benefit although they didn't particularly bother me. (Magnets were covered in detail earlier.) If you want to check out something along this line which is supposed to offer a foot massage as well as magnetic therapy, you can order "**Pressure Point Insoles**" from Starcrest of California (1-909-657-2793). They are certainly inexpensive—$3 a pair! (I did a double take when I saw that price in their ad.)

There is one other category of shoe inserts which kind of fall in between the arch-and-foot-support devices and the Dr. Scholl type cushion pads. These are exemplified by **Spenco** brand insoles which are full shoe length and made with polyurethane bonded to a soft material. The Spencos have contoured heel cups and arch supports and sell for about $20 a pair. I use them in New Balance running shoes from which I removed the original insoles. The Spencos seem to do a good job in the shock absorbing area and appear to keep your feet aligned properly.

3. Socks

For greater foot comfort PNers agree socks should be **soft**, **thick** and maybe a **little loose**. Also they should be made without seams and of non-irritating materials. The Mayo Clinic suggests the best ones are 100% cotton.

One PNer says **Thorlo** socks are the only ones he'll wear. The company which makes them claims they have a patented system of high-density padding in the ball and heel which gives protection against impacts and absorbs shocks. Thorlos are available in many sporting good stores at $5.95 a pair.

Another PNer mentions socks which are said to be designed especially for those with diabetes or other circulation problems. They are available for $5.99 a pair from a Florida outfit called the Sugar Free Marketplace (1-800-726-6191). Made of cotton, they have what Sugar Free calls a "full heel and toe and low profile seam to reduce the risk of irritation." They come in a variety of sizes and colors for both men and women.

4. General Foot Care

Good foot care is important, particularly for people with diabetic neuropathy. Feet and toes should be checked daily for cuts, bruises and infections. Sometimes it may be necessary to use a mirror to do this properly. People with diabetes should also wash their feet daily with warm water and a mild soap. Since these PNers tend to sweat less than most people they should also consider regularly applying a moisturizer to help prevent dry and cracked skin. Most importantly, their shoes should always be examined before they are put on to make sure the shoes have no tears or hidden objects which might cause foot injury.

Special Considerations—Hands

The natural progression of the obnoxious malady we suffer is frequently from our feet to our hands. A number of things can be done, though, to make you more comfortable if you are such an afflicted PNer.

Perhaps the first point is to keep your hands **warm** when nerves begin to act up, particularly if you've just come in from the outside where it was cold. Other than to soak your hands in warm water, **gloves** are the obvious answer here when things get really bad. One PNer mentions something called **Hand Cuffs** available from JC Penney. They are built into a sweatshirt and can be rolled up or pulled down to your finger tips as desired. Some PNers have used **thermal socks** over their hands at night while others wear **arthritic gloves** made of spandex material through the wee hours.

Hand exercises also help. A squeeze ball works well

and even wringing out a wet wash cloth repeatedly will limber your hands and often make them feel better.

Other Ways to Cope

PNers are inventive and a number of them have devised different ways to make each day more tolerable. Here's a list of things I've heard or read about:

1. Buy a cane that folds out into a little stool—you'll find it particularly useful when you're waiting in check-out lines.
2. Install shower bars or shower chairs to keep you from a bad fall, and a raised toilet seat—PNers usually don't have the same sense of balance as we used to.
3. Get some long foot and bath brushes.
4. Try zippers rather than buttons on clothing and a tool called "Zip-it" when even zippers cause problems.
5. Get light weight dressing sticks which help you put on clothes and molded sock aids to help in slipping on socks.
6. Buy extra long shoe horns—they come up to 36" long.
7. Use Velcro instead of shoe laces for easy closures and releases, or elastic shoe laces, as well as for other clothing items.
8. Invest in a vibration foot massager you could keep

under the desk or where you read—for a "quick fix" foot reliever.

9. If your hands cause you difficulty in writing, make your pen or pencil "fatter" by sliding a foam rubber curler over them or buy a special adapter.

10. Use double handled cups and pots which are easier to hold.

11. Place pieces of Dycem—a high-friction material available at medical supply houses—on kitchen surfaces to keep things from sliding—e.g., while you're opening cans.

12. Get meat cutters which can be operated with one hand.

13. Buy grip knobs for turning on faucets and plastic turning handles for doorknobs.

14. Use scooters at grocery stores and malls—don't let your pride get in the way of making shopping more manageable.

15. If you need a walker consider one called the "Maddak"—it's adjustable and lightweight.

16. Obtain a handicap parking placard or sticker. (If your feet are keeping you away from the stores, restaurants or theaters, you're as much entitled to them as anyone. You'll need your doctor's okay, though.)[3]

17. Get up and walk around occasionally when you've

---

[3] I agree with what one PNer said (though I don't have handicap placards myself): "My PN disease is just as disabling as any other handicap. The spaces are for folks with a handicap and believe me, my PN is a handicap!"

been sitting for a long while—it helps to get blood down to the feet.

18. Try swimming fins called "Zoomers" which reportedly help ward off neck and shoulder pains while swimming (from WorldWide Aquatics at 1-800-726-1530).

19. For pain in your forearms buy lightweight wristbands to be worn below the elbow—available from sporting goods departments at Wal-Mart for about a dollar.

20. Take off your shoes every once in a while, wiggle your toes and let your feet enjoy the day same as you—they'll thank you for it. While you're at it give them both a little massage. They'll be *doubly* pleased.

21. If your feet are particularly bothering you (so what else is new) try wrapping an Ace bandage around them through the arch to see if that helps (need I add one at a time and not together?). Perhaps it's like an orthotic in effect, which seems to benefit some PNers.

22. Make a cup of "sleepy-time" (caffeine-free) tea or drink a glass of warm milk before you go to bed.

23. Try eating small, frequent meals and avoiding fats if your stomach empties slowly, indicating gastroparesis.

24. Move to a warmer climate if you're able to—probably only makes sense if you have other reasons but some PNers who have done so are sure it's helped ease their symptoms.

25. Buy a soft cover book—*We Are Not Alone—Learning to Live With Chronic Illness* (S. K. Pitzele 1986, Workman Publishing), for about $10—it's full of ideas on adaptive aids and contains a comprehensive listing of merchants selling handy devices for easier living.

Another reminder. Join the **Neuropathy Association** if you haven't already! You can greatly benefit from the on-line comradeship found in their bulletin board and in their chat groups, sharing common frustrations and learning from each other. As somebody said, you'll be reminded over and over that you're not in this all by yourself. That realization can itself be powerful medicine! The Association can be reached at 1-800-247-6968 or at their web site: www.neuropathy.org.

Incidentally, another important organization that PNers should join is the Neuropathy Trust. It also is an excellent source of information and support for people affected by peripheral neuropathy. Though based in the United Kingdom, the Trust reaches out to people living in many parts of the world. Additionally, the Trust is actively working with pharmaceutical companies in the UK to foster the development of other treatment approaches to PN. These efforts are similar to those of the Neuropathy Association in the United States. The Trust web site is www.neuropathy-trust.org.

Final Notes

Just reading many of the patient comments, particularly in the third and fourth chapters, should give anybody a sense of the frustration, desperation and even hopelessness that some PNers are going through. Those who attend these victims, or at least are around them much, need to understand the devastating psychological as well as physical impacts that neuropathies can have on lives. I hope the book helps on that.

It is important for all to understand, though, that "impacts" are experienced both ways. **Caregivers**, whether spouses or other family members, can suffer greatly as well as the care receivers, not only from seeing the pain and agony their loved ones are going through but also from sheer exhaustion in performing their own caregiving responsibilities! **Patience** and **understanding** by each party for what the other is facing are essential.

Incidentally, there is an organization devoted to the special needs of caregivers with an Internet web site: **www.caregivers.com**. Also there is an Internet chat room for those caregivers who take care of patients with **neurological disorders**. It's held on Thursday evenings at 8 P. M. Eastern time and sponsored by the

Department of Neurology at Massachusetts General Hospital. The web address is: **http://neuro-www.mgh. harvard.edu**. (You will also find a forum there for peripheral neuropathy. Are you maybe getting the idea that having access to the Internet is important for PNers and those around them? It may not be indispensable but it sure helps.) An excellent book for caregivers is offered by the Visiting Nurse Associations of America: *Caregiver's Handbook*, DK Publishing Company, 1998. It offers many good ideas on how a caregiver can take care of a patient properly as well as how the caretaking experience itself can be managed and survived! It's available for under $15.

Speaking of patient comments, you really have to admire the generosity of so many PNers in sharing their experiences with others. Until a "cure" for peripheral neuropathy, or something very close to it, comes along we need to learn from each other what helps and what doesn't. Which brings me back to the Neuropathy Association. One of their principal goals is to promote research into effective treatments for PN. Join the association and make things **happen** with the help of your contributions!

I think by now you've seen how rapidly things are changing in the matter of peripheral neuropathy treatments. There seems to be an accelerating flow of data from clinical studies and other sources on medications and alternative treatment approaches. For example, there is new information all the time on vitamin, herb and other nutrient therapy. At the back of the book there is a form which you can use to indicate your interest in obtaining ongoing current information concerning these subjects. If you will give us your name and address on that form and return it to us, we will see that you are kept current on our up-date plans.

*   *   *

I think I've finally figured out what works for me with this crazy stuff. There are a lot of acronyms in this book and I'll add one more—**BEND**. It stands for **B** complex vitamins, **E**xercise, **N**eurontin and **D**iet. If I keep on BENDing I'm sure I'll make it. Try some of the things mentioned here yourself and make up your own word- and routine- with the help of your doctor. Maybe something like **MEET** (**M**agnets, **E**lavil, **E**xercise—always gotta do that if you can—and **T**ouch). I'm going to MEET and **BEAT** (**B**aclofen, **E**xercise, **A**mitriptyline and **T**ramadol anyone?) this problem I've got with these worthless, no-good feet of mine! Or try **QUIET** (**Q**igong, **U**ltram, **I**mipramine, **E**xercise and **T**ENS). I'm going to QUIET down my popping nerves. You get the idea. It's corny but it'll keep you focused.

Index

Index

Index

Index

Index

Index

Index

Index

Announcing Two New Books on Peripheral Neuropathy!

Since the book you have in your hands, *Numb Toes and Aching Soles: Coping with Peripheral Neuropathy,* was first published in July 1999, its author, John Senneff, has written two new books on this painful, debilitating disorder:

Numb Toes and Others Woes: More on Peripheral Neuropathy, was initially published in July 2001. In the same reader-friendly style of his first book the author here

- examines the nature of neuropathic pain in depth
- updates studies on the efficacy of various drugs
- reports on novel treatment approaches such as nerve regeneration and cellular therapies (including gene therapy, stem cell technology, "biologic mini-pumps," and nerve cell disablement)
- discusses promising new drugs awaiting government approvals, and
- describes unusual neuropathies, best ways of working with doctors, and new sources of patient assistance.

John Senneff's latest book, *Nutrients for Neuropathy,* came out in July 2002. It is full of clinical studies and references concerning an especially important treatment option. Everything is covered in this science-based, easy-reading guide to natural healing including

- most bio-available nutrient supplement forms
- suggested dosages and best times to take
- safe upper limits and possible drug interactions
- valuable comments from experts, and
- a specific nutrient supplement program

All of our *Numb Toes* books have received strong endorsements from both patients and medical professionals and are sold all over the world.

If you are interested in being current on the various ways of overcoming the ravages of peripheral neuropathy, either using conventional medical methods or pursuing more natural alternatives, we strongly urge you to buy these two books. Look for them at your favorite bookstore. If not available there they may be ordered directly from the publisher on one of the Book Order forms that follow this page. (You may also order additional copies of this book for friends, family members, and others there as well.)

Visit us at *www.medpress.com* for more on *Numb Toes* books!

BOOK ORDER FORM

Order extra copies for any friends or relatives you think might benefit – even for your doctor!)

Telephone orders: Call 1-888-MED-9898 toll free (1-888-633-9898)
Fax orders: Fax the form you have filled in below to 1-902-492-0013
Postal orders: Mail the form you have filled in below to:

    MedPress/Origin BioMed, PO Box 81,

    Halifax, Nova Scotia, Canada B3J 2L4

Please send me the following:

    Nutrients for Neuropathy

      _____ copies (paperback), $22.95 each

    Numb Toes and Aching Soles: Coping with Peripheral Neuropathy

      _____ copies (paperback), $24.95 each

      _____ copies (professional case bound edition), $29.95 each

    Numb Toes and Other Woes: More on Peripheral Neuropathy

      _____ copies (paperback), $24.95 each

      _____ copies (professional case bound edition), $29.95 each

Shipping & Handling

    Please add for U.S. deliveries, $7 for first book, $3 for each additional book. For shipments outside the U.S., please call 1-888-633-9898 or email orders@medpress.com for information.

Payment: _____ Check (payable to "MedPress")

         _____ Credit Card:
         The undersigned hereby consents to payment for orders to be charged to a credit card listed below:

Authorised Signature: _____

Print Name on Card: _____

Exp Date: _____

Credit Card Number: _____

Card Type: Visa___ Mastercard___ AMEX___

3-Digit Code (req'd): _____

Corresponding Address for Credit Card: _____

_____

Corresponding Telephone Number for Credit Card: _____

BOOK ORDER FORM

Order extra copies for any friends or relatives you think might benefit – even for your doctor!)

Telephone orders: Call 1-888-MED-9898 toll free (1-888-633-9898)
Fax orders: Fax the form you have filled in below to 1-902-492-0013
Postal orders: Mail the form you have filled in below to:
> *MedPress/Origin BioMed, PO Box 81,*
> *Halifax, Nova Scotia, Canada B3J 2L4*

Please send me the following:
> *Nutrients for Neuropathy*
> _____ copies (paperback), $22.95 each
> *Numb Toes and Aching Soles: Coping with Peripheral Neuropathy*
> _____ copies (paperback), $24.95 each
> _____ copies (professional case bound edition), $29.95 each
> *Numb Toes and Other Woes: More on Peripheral Neuropathy*
> _____ copies (paperback), $24.95 each
> _____ copies (professional case bound edition), $29.95 each

Shipping & Handling
> Please add for U.S. deliveries, $7 for first book, $3 for each additional book. For shipments outside the U.S., please call 1-888-633-9898 or email orders@medpress.com for information.

Payment: _____ Check (payable to "MedPress")

_____ Credit Card:
The undersigned hereby consents to payment for orders to be charged to a credit card listed below:

Authorised Signature: _____

Print Name on Card: _____

Exp Date: _____

Credit Card Number: _____

Card Type: Visa____ Mastercard____ AMEX____

3-Digit Code (req'd): _____

Corresponding Address for Credit Card: _____

_____

Corresponding Telephone Number for Credit Card: _____

BOOK ORDER FORM

Order extra copies for any friends or relatives you think might benefit – even for your doctor!)

Telephone orders: Call 1-888-MED-9898 toll free (1-888-633-9898)
Fax orders: Fax the form you have filled in below to 1-902-492-0013
Postal orders: Mail the form you have filled in below to:
> *MedPress / Origin BioMed, PO Box 81,*
> *Halifax, Nova Scotia, Canada B3J 2L4*

Please send me the following:
> *Nutrients for Neuropathy*
> _____ copies (paperback), $22.95 each
> *Numb Toes and Aching Soles: Coping with Peripheral Neuropathy*
> _____ copies (paperback), $24.95 each
> _____ copies (professional case bound edition), $29.95 each
> *Numb Toes and Other Woes: More on Peripheral Neuropathy*
> _____ copies (paperback), $24.95 each
> _____ copies (professional case bound edition), $29.95 each

Shipping & Handling
> Please add for U.S. deliveries, $7 for first book, $3 for each additional
> book. For shipments outside the U.S., please call 1-888-633-9898
> or email orders@medpress.com for information.

Payment: _____ Check (payable to "MedPress")

_____ Credit Card:
The undersigned hereby consents to payment for orders
to be charged to a credit card listed below:

Authorised Signature: _____

Print Name on Card: _____

Exp Date: _____

Credit Card Number: _____

Card Type: Visa___ Mastercard___ AMEX___

3-Digit Code (req'd): _____

Corresponding Address for Credit Card: _____
_____

Corresponding Telephone Number for Credit Card: _____